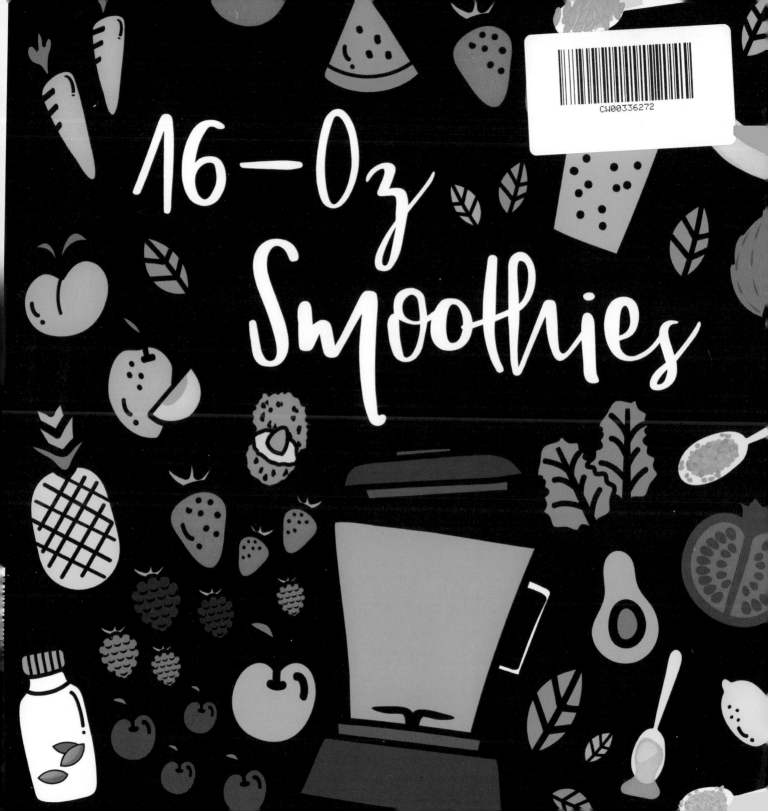

16-Oz Smoothies

FOLLOW US:

 youtube.com/cookmenot

 instagram.com/cookmenotrecipes

 tenor.com/users/cookmenotrecipes

 www.zazzle.com/store/cookmenotrecipes

 https://www.etsy.com/shop/cookmenot

Contents

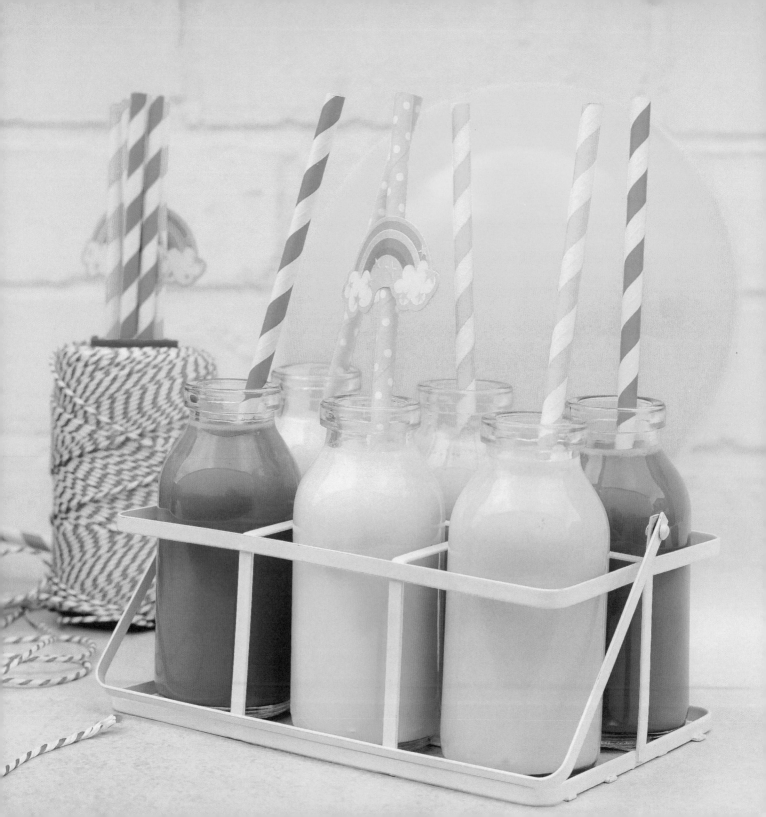

Introduction

Many people find it difficult to pack whole fruits and vegetables, healthy fats, and antioxidant-rich protein into a single meal. The smoothie is a drink that quickly combines these ingredients without a significant increase in calorie intake--all while retaining essential vitamins, minerals, and fiber.

16-Oz Smoothies is a book of 30 doodle-style recipes--that's 30 tasty and nutritious meals. For anyone who wants to nourish the body, hydrates the skin, protect against diseases, lose weight, reduce inflammation, detox and cleanse, boost immunity, or snack fast after working out or being on the go, smoothies give real energy and are a nice caffeine replacement. Even better: smoothies don't cause bloat and gently supply the body with a daily dose of all your necessary nutrients.

Some notes about these recipes: By using frozen fruit, there is no need to add ice in most recipes, which can water down smoothies. Sugar and artificial sweeteners are not used or recommended for these recipes. Fruits are naturally sweet, but you can sweeten some recipes with honey or maple syrup.

These smoothie recipes serve about 16 ounces. Feel free to freeze the leftover portion for later or get creative and make frozen popsicles with them.

We hope these easy-to-make smoothie recipes bring you great health, glowing skin, and a tasty experience. Feel free to adjust these recipes to fit your health's needs and personal preference.

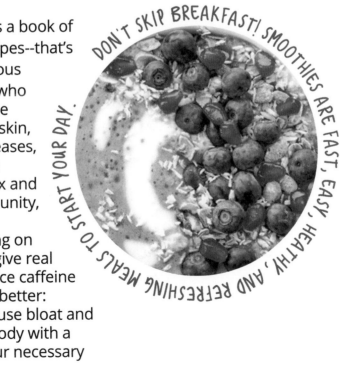

DON'T SKIP BREAKFAST! SMOOTHIES ARE FAST, EASY, HEALTHY, AND REFRESHING MEALS TO START YOUR DAY.

Basic Anatomy of Smoothie

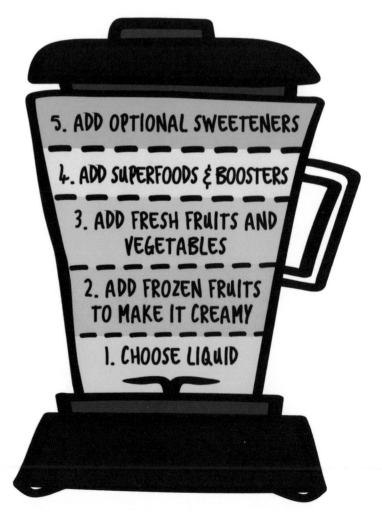

5. ADD OPTIONAL SWEETENERS

4. ADD SUPERFOODS & BOOSTERS

3. ADD FRESH FRUITS AND VEGETABLES

2. ADD FROZEN FRUITS TO MAKE IT CREAMY

1. CHOOSE LIQUID

The 4 Herbs

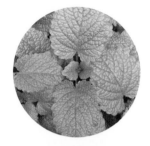

Mint : This invigorating herb helps lower toxin buildup in our stomach and colon when improper digestion, constipation, and bloating take place.

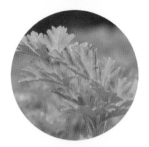

Parsley : With fresh distinctive flavor, parsley helps the bladder, kidneys, and liver remove toxins out of our bodies.

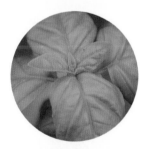

Basil : This popular herb not only adds warm flavor but also helps reduce inflammation, strengthen kidneys, and provide anti-aging and antibacterial properties.

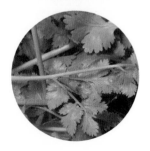

Cilantro : With refreshing citrusy flavor, this sweet herb has an ability to bind to toxic heavy metals and extract them from our bodies.

Superfoods Boosters

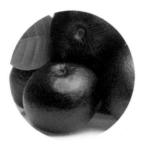

Acai Berry: Loaded with nutrients and antioxidants, these small purple berries help prevent early signs of aging and skin regeneration. Studies have found that the berry improves memory and focus. It is also known for stabilizing blood sugar level, improving digestion, detoxifying the liver and kidneys, and controlling appetite.

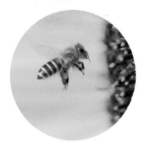

Bee Pollen: Regarded as one of nature's most nourishing foods, bee pollen contains nearly all nutrients required by humans. Half of its protein is in the form of free amino acids that are ready to be used directly by the body for such benefits as hormone balance and detox. Bee pollen can have a significant impact on the health of one's immune system. It contains vitamins B, C, D, and E, as well as calcium, magnesium, selenium, cysteine, and a variety of proteins.

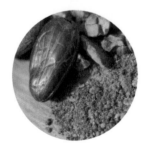

Cacao: With 40 times the antioxidants of blueberries, the health benefits of raw cacao are fantastic for your entire body. It can improve memory, reduce heart disease, shed fat, increase immunity, boost your bliss, and give energize you.

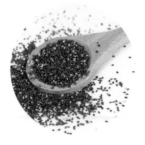

Chia Seeds: As a staple in Mayan and Aztec diets for centuries, these tiny seeds are an excellent source of omega-3 fatty acids, rich in antioxidants, fiber, iron, and calcium. Omega-3 fatty acids help raise HDL cholesterol, the "good" cholesterol that protects against heart disease, stroke, cancer, and diabetes.

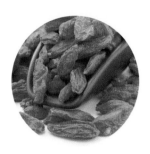

Goji Berries : Known as the anti-aging fruit, these native-to-china red berries are a darling of the superfood world. Packed with powerful antioxidants, they benefit the skin, vision, and immune system. They also balance hormones and prevent and fight cancer.

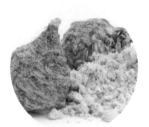

Maca Root : This adaptogen, which is often compared to ginseng, relieves pain, treats anemia, balances hormone, addresses low libido, and lessens symptoms of menopause. Though the herb itself does not contain any hormones, is made up of nutrients that are essential to support normal hormone production. It supports the hypothalamus and the pituitary gland which are the "master glands" of the body that regulate a network of other glands to do a host of things, including keeping us in homeostasis, regulating our metabolisms, and controlling cortisol, and stimulating sperm production and maturation eggs in ovaries.

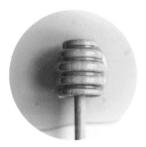

Manuka Honey : From its skin benefits to its antibacterial properties, there's a lot to love about this honey. It is used for reducing inflammation of stomach and intestines, defending against infections, and supporting digestive health.

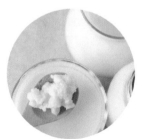

Probiotics : This good bacteria helps improve digestion, aid in proper nutrient absorption, boost the immune system, and help with overall well-being.

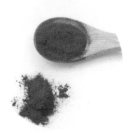

Spirulina : This nutrient-dense algae helps alkalizing your green smoothie, increase energy, boost immunity, and flush heavy metals and toxins from the body.

Plant-Based Protein

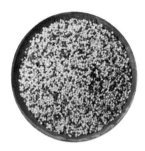

Quinoa: This gluten-free whole grain is high in protein and contains all nine essential amino acids. It is high in fiber, magnesium, B-vitamins, iron, potassium, calcium, phosphorus, manganese, vitamin E, and antioxidants. Benefits include weight loss, improved heart health, detoxification of the body, and improved digestive health. Quinoa also helps in regulating diabetes and reducing gallstones.

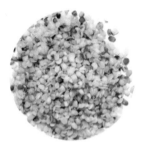

Hemp Hearts: These nutty seeds contain easily digested proteins, balanced 3:1 omega-3 and omega-6 fatty acids, Gamma Linolenic Acid (GLA), antioxidants, essential amino acids, soluble fiber, iron, zinc, carotene, phospholipids, phytosterols, vitamin B1, vitamin B2, vitamin B6, vitamin D, vitamin E, chlorophyll, calcium, magnesium, sulfur, and copper. Hemp seeds are good for digestion, the heart, hormone health, and hair, skin, and nails.

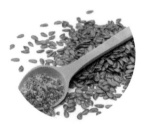

Ground Flaxseeds: Loaded with nutrients, these seeds are rich sources of omega-3 fatty acid and Lignans. Their proven health benefits are lowering risk of stroke, preventing cancer, lowering blood sugar level, and improving brain health.

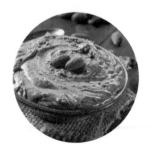

Almond Butter: A small serving of almond butter contains a generous amount of magnesium, which helps balance blood sugar level and boosts heart health by promoting the flow of blood and oxygen.

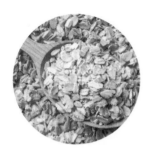

Rolled Oats: Containing both soluble beta-glucan and insoluble fiber, these nutritious grains help reduce cholesterol and blood sugar levels, promotes healthy gut bacteria, and increases feelings of fullness. Whole oats are rich in antioxidants, including Avenanthramides.

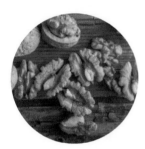

Walnuts: Containing a number of neuroprotective compounds, vitamin E, folate, copper, manganese, melatonin, and antioxidants, these nuts are an excellent source of anti-inflammatory omega-3 essential fatty acids -- in the form of alpha-linolenic acid (ALA). Several clinical studies have shown walnuts have potential in preventing neurodegenerative conditions such as Parkinson's and Alzheimer's disease, cancer, and heart disease, in addition to promoting weight loss and maintaining brain health. These nuts can also help reduce the risk of type 2 diabetes.

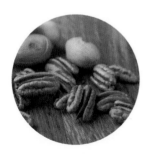

Pecans: Loaded with vitamins and minerals such as manganese, copper, potassium, calcium, iron, magnesium, zinc, and selenium, these delicious nuts have more flavonoids — a type of antioxidant found mostly in veggies and fruit — than any other tree nut. People who eat diets high in flavonoids are less likely to develop chronic diseases, such as heart disease, diabetes, some cancers, and cognitive decline. Not only do they contain very little sugar, but pecans may also help improve blood sugar levels overall by slowing down the rate of absorption from the bloodstream into peripheral tissues.

Healthy Fat Boosters

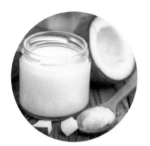

Coconut Oil : High in natural saturated fats, this wonder oil benefits can improve skin, hair, digestion, and boosting immunity. Coconut oil can promote weight loss and treat yeast infections, too. The lauric acid present in coconut oil helps in preventing various heart problems like high LDL "bad" cholesterol levels and high blood pressure. It also promotes the effective utilization of blood glucose, which prevents and treats diabetes.

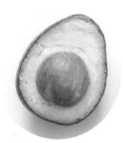

Avocado : This incredibly nutritious fruit is extremely low in cholesterol and sugar. It is a good source of monounsaturated fatty acids, which promotes a healthy heart. It also helps nourish the skin with essential vitamins and keep your eyes healthy against cataracts, eye diseases related to age, and macular degeneration.

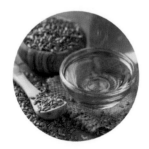

Flaxseed Oil : High in omega-3 fatty acids, health benefits of this oil includes its ability to improve heart health, reduce inflammation and gout, and prevent cancer and premature aging. It also helps boost the immune system and regulate digestion. Flaxseed oil helps regulate hormones in post-menopausal women. It lowers blood pressure, prevents various gastrointestinal diseases, and improves eye health.

Spice Boosters

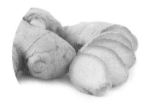 **Ginger** : This fresh spice helps reduce gas, nausea, and body inflammation.

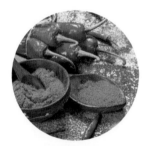 **Ground Red Pepper** : With distinctive flavor, this herb helps the bladder, kidneys, and liver remove toxins from the body.

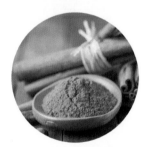 **Cinnamon** : Cinnamon not only adds warm flavor but also help reduce inflammation, strengthen kidneys, and provide anti-aging and antibacterial properties.

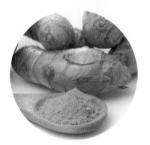 **Turmeric** : With citrusy flavor, turmeric can bind to toxic heavy metals and draw them out of our bodies.

Washing Fruits & Vegetables

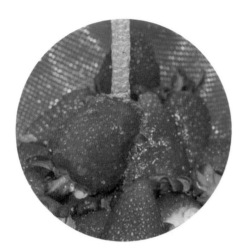

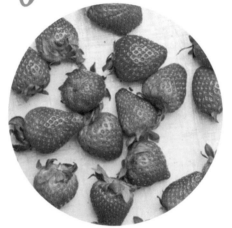

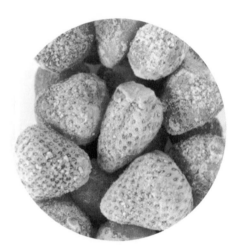

STEP 1: WASH

Spray cleanser on the surface of fruit or vegetable and rinse well with warm water

STEP 2: DRY

Wipe the fruit or vegetable with paper towels and leave it outside until dry

STEP 3: FREEZE

Freeze in a glass container

14

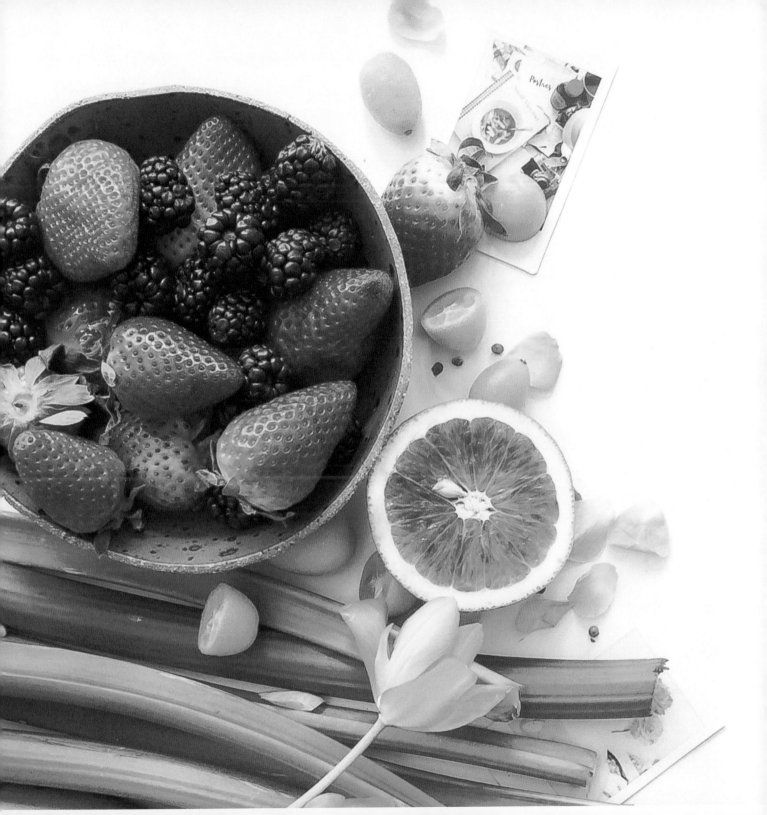

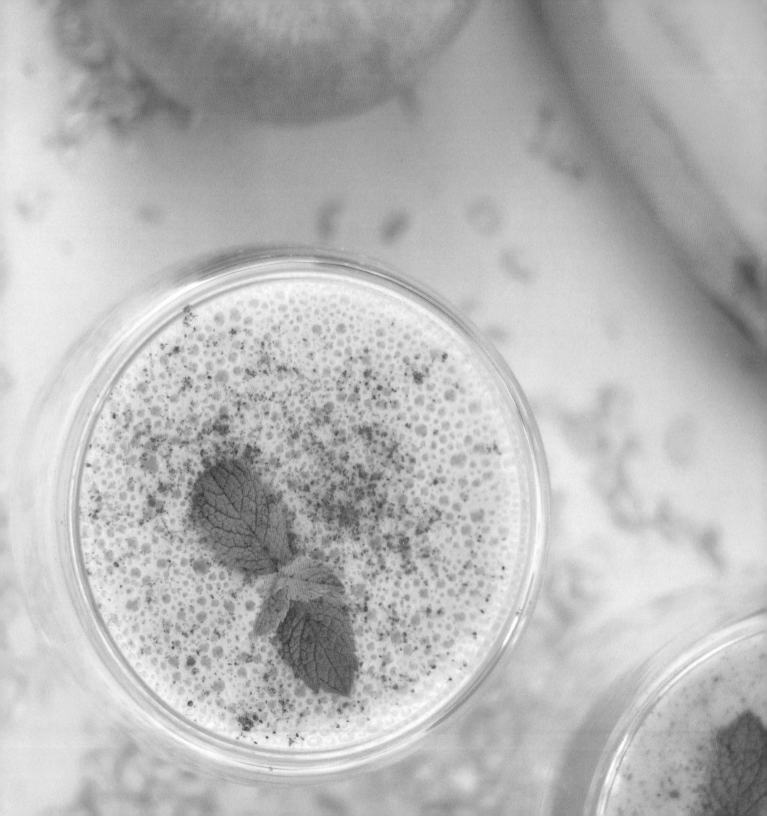

Chapter 1:

Morning Meals

Rise & Shine

Ingredients:

1 Cup **Orange Juice**

1/4 Cup **Greek-Style Almond Milk Yogurt (Vanilla Flavor)**

1 Cup **Frozen Mangoes**

1/2 Cup **Shredded Carrots**

2 Tbsp **Hemp Hearts**

1/2 tsp **Manuka Honey**

NOTE: WE PREFER MAKING ORANGE JUICE FROM SCRATCH OVER STORE-BOUGHT.

HIGH VITAMIN C

Loaded with vitamin C, this refreshing smoothie is nutritious and collagen-boosting. It's a great go-to breakfast.

Instructions:

1. Place ingredients in a blender and purée until it is smooth and creamy.

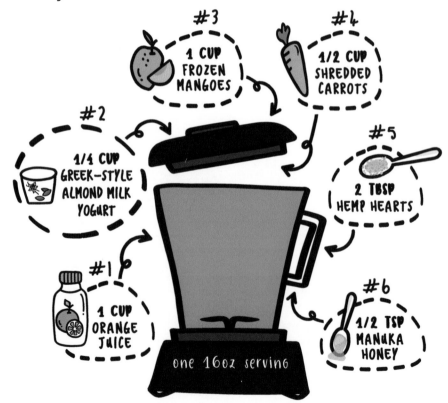

2. Pour into glass, garnish with fresh mango or berries, and serve immediately.

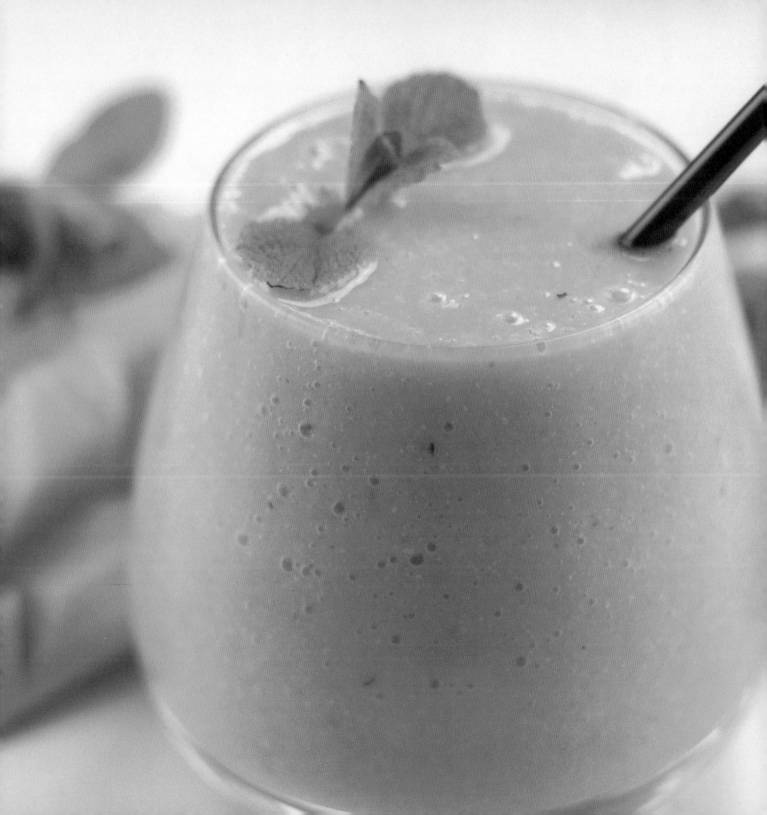

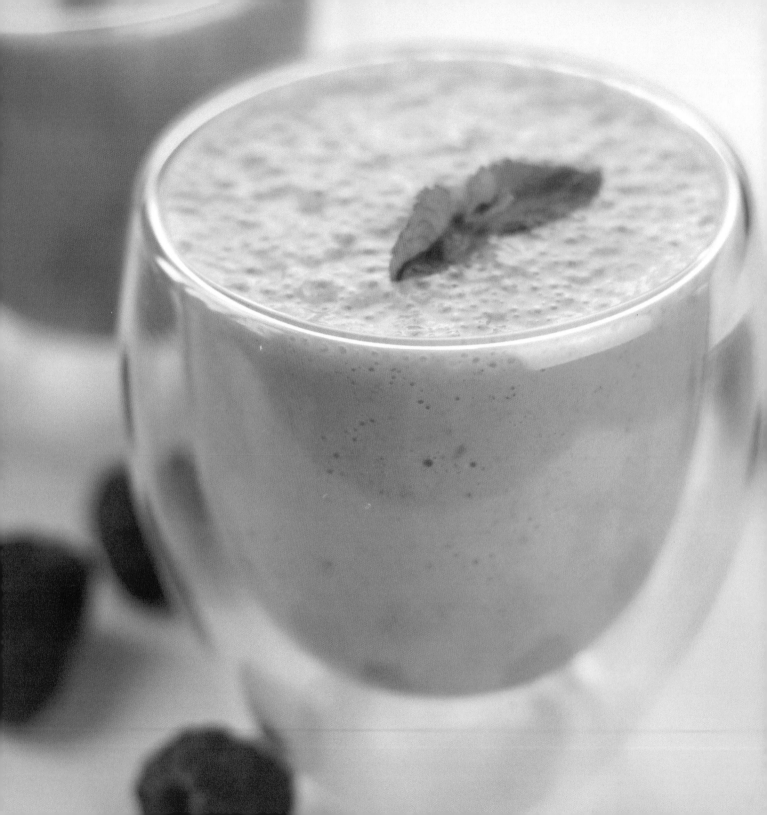

Ruby Boost

Loaded with antioxidants, this refreshing smoothie additional raspberries makes it nutritious and delightfully red.

Instructions:

1. Place ingredients in a blender and purée until smooth and creamy.

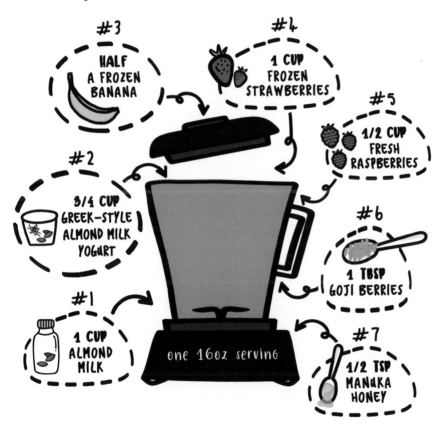

2. Pour into glass, garnish with fresh strawberries, and pomegranate seeds, and serve immediately.

Ingredients:

1 Cup **Almond Milk**

3/4 Cup **Greek-Style Almond Milk Yogurt (Vanilla Flavor)**

1/2 **A Frozen Banana**

1 Cup **Frozen Strawberries**

1/2 Cup **Fresh Raspberries**

1 Tbsp **Goji Berries**

1/2 tsp **Manuka Honey**

HIGH ANTIOXIDANTS

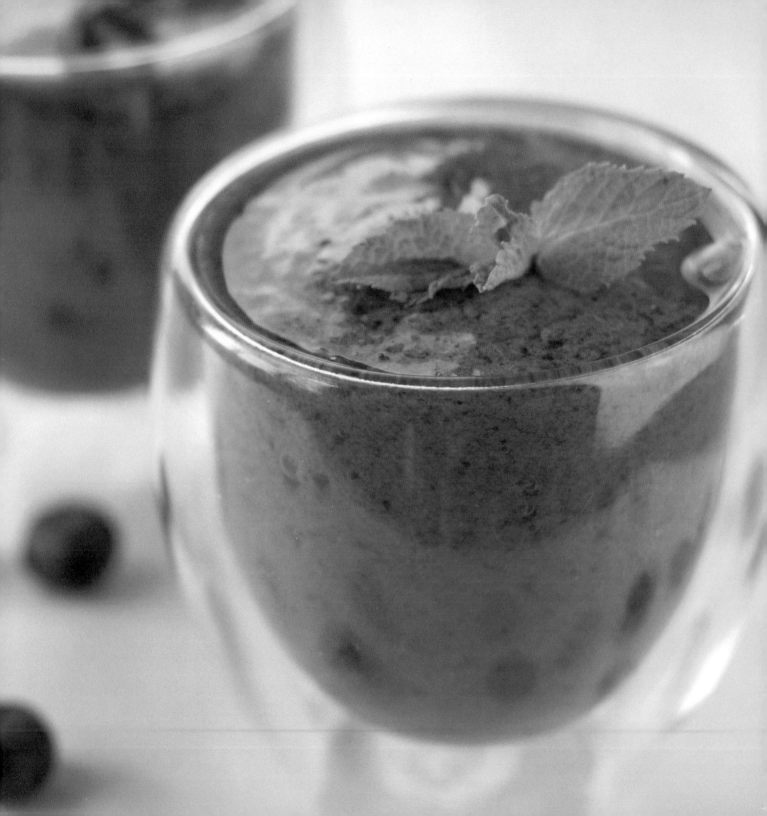

Mixed Berries

This antioxidant and nutrient-dense smoothie is not only a delicious treat but also an energizing breakfast.

Instructions:

1. Place ingredients in a blender and purée until smooth and creamy.

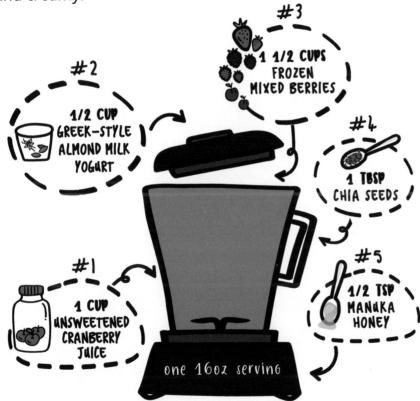

#3
1 1/2 CUPS FROZEN MIXED BERRIES

#2
1/2 CUP GREEK-STYLE ALMOND MILK YOGURT

#4
1 TBSP CHIA SEEDS

#1
1 CUP UNSWEETENED CRANBERRY JUICE

#5
1/2 TSP MANUKA HONEY

one 16oz serving

2. Pour into glass, garnish with fresh berries and goji berries, and serve immediately.

Ingredients:

1 Cup **Unsweetened Cranberry Juice**

1/2 Cup **Greek-Style Almond Milk Yogurt (Vanilla Flavor)**

1 1/2 Cup **Frozen Mixed Berries**

1 Tbsp **Chia Seeds**

1/2 tsp **Manuka Honey**

Fresh berries and goji berries, for serving

HIGH ANTIOXIDANTS

23

Blueberry Oatmeal

Ingredients:

1 Cup **Almond Milk**

1/2 Cup **Greek-Style Almond Milk Yogurt (Vanilla Flavor)**

1/2 **A Frozen Banana**

1 Cup **Frozen Blueberries**

2 Tbsp **Rolled Oats**

1 tsp **Maple Syrup**

With its high antioxidants, Magnesium, and fiber, this nutritious smoothie will get you up and running with high energy.

Instructions:

1. Place ingredients in a blender and purée until it is smooth and creamy.

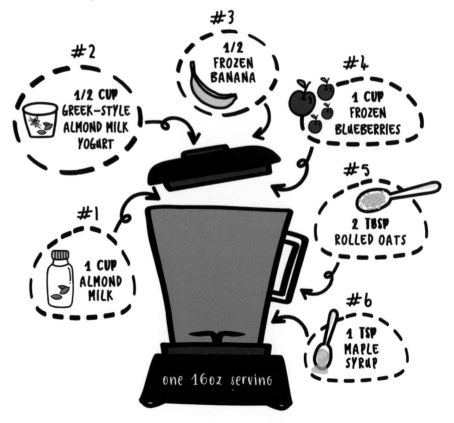

#2 1/2 CUP GREEK-STYLE ALMOND MILK YOGURT

#3 1/2 FROZEN BANANA

#4 1 CUP FROZEN BLUEBERRIES

#5 2 TBSP ROLLED OATS

#1 1 CUP ALMOND MILK

#6 1 TSP MAPLE SYRUP

one 16oz serving

2. Pour into glass, garnish with fresh banana, and serve immediately.

LOW SUGAR

24

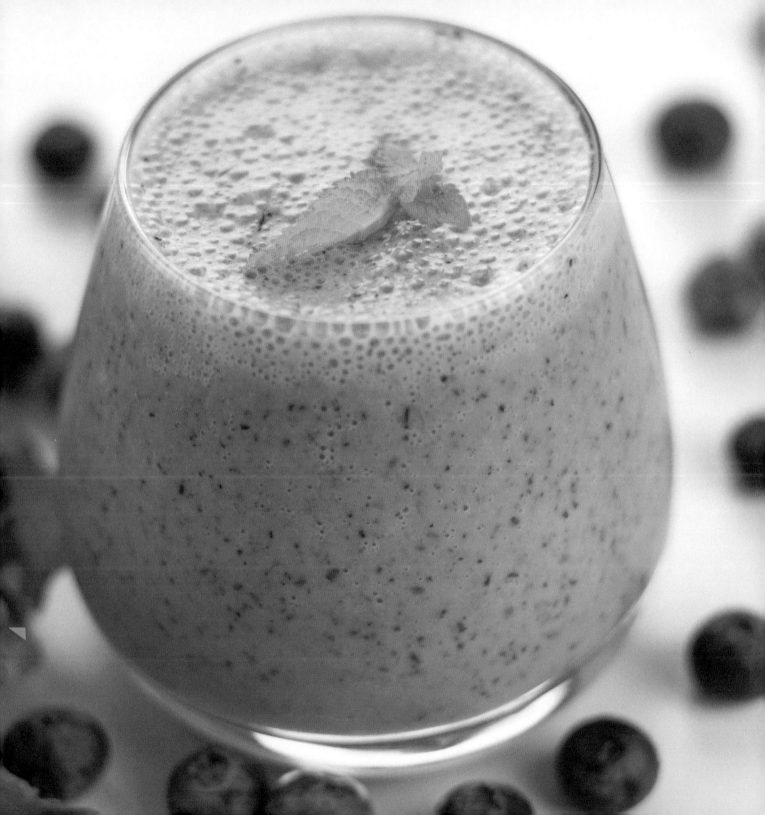

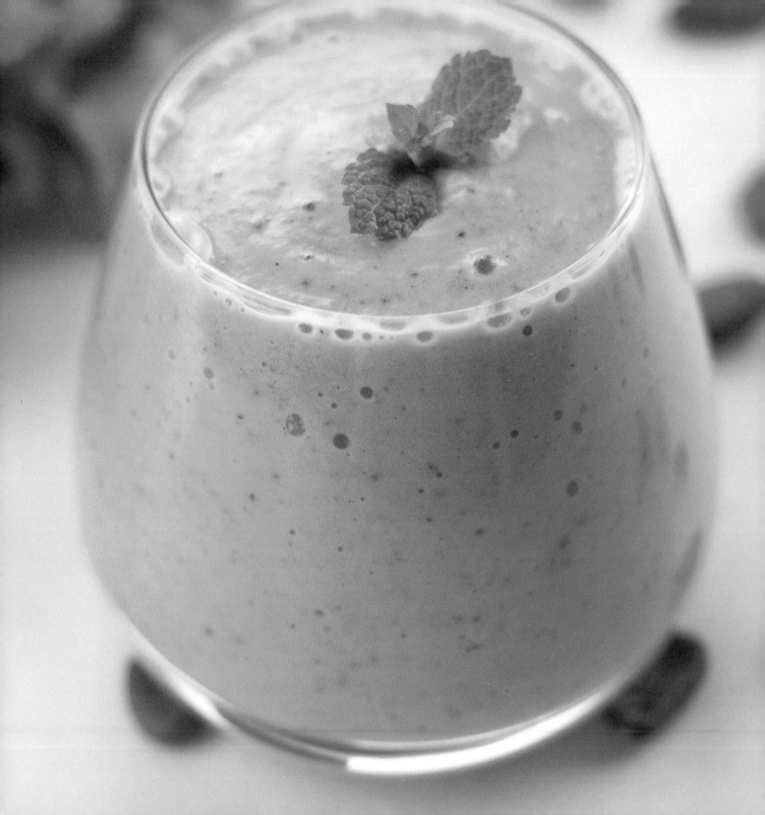

Cacao Mint

With minty flavor, this cacao smoothie is not only a delicious creamy treat for breakfast or snack time, but also loaded with nutrients.

Instructions:

1. Place ingredients in a blender and purée until it is smooth.

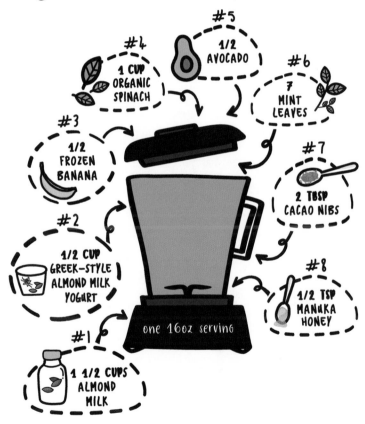

2. Pour into glass and serve immediately.

Ingredients:

1 1/2 Cups **Almond Milk**

1/2 Cup **Greek-Style Almond Milk Yogurt (Plain or Vanilla Flavor)**

1/2 **Frozen Banana**

1 Cup **Organic Spinach**

1/2 **Avocado**

7 **Mint Leaves**

2 Tbsp **Cacao Nibs**

1/2 tsp **Manuka Honey**

HIGH ANTIOXIDANTS

Apple Oatmeal

Loaded with vitamin C and fiber, this smoothie is a comforting energy boost to start your day.

Ingredients:

1 Cup **Almond Milk**

1/4 Cup **Greek-Style Almond Milk Yogurt (Plain or Vanilla Flavor)**

1/2 **Frozen Banana**

1 Cup **Organic Green Apple Slices**

2 Tbsp **Rolled Oats**

1 tsp **Maple Syrup**

A Few Sprinkles **Ground Cinnamon**

Banana slices or fresh berries, for serving

28

Instructions:

1. Place ingredients in a blender and purée until it is smooth.

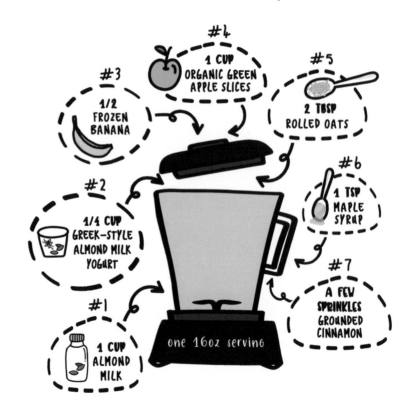

2. Pour into glass, garnish with sliced banana or fresh berries, and serve immediately.

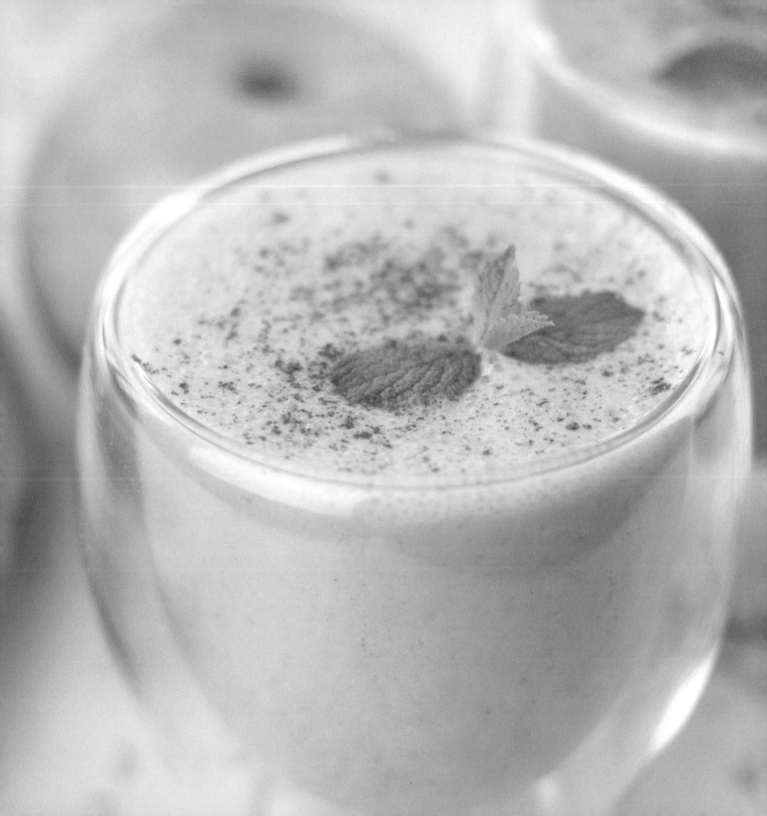

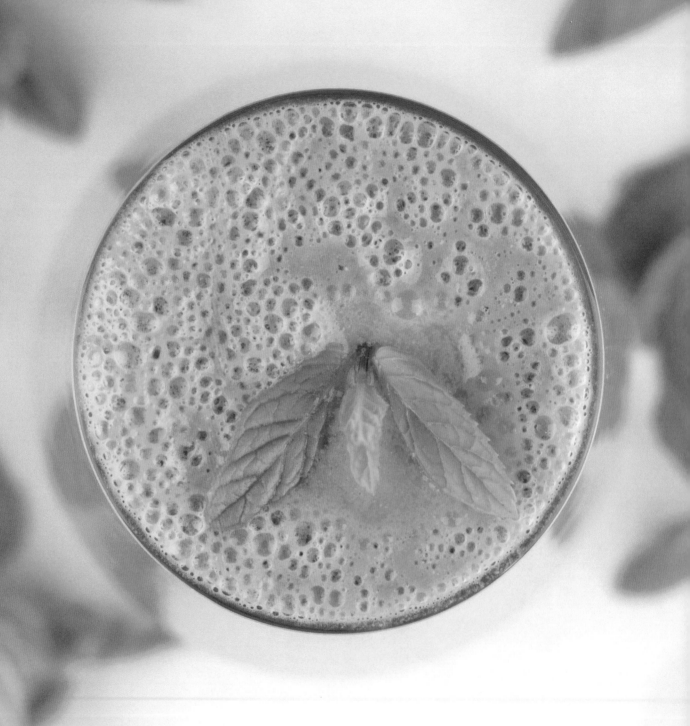

Chapter 2:

Ohhh, so green!

Matcha Green

Ingredients:

1 Cup **Coconut Water**

1/2 Cup **Greek-Style Almond Milk Yogurt (Plain or Vanilla Flavor)**

3/4 Cup **Frozen Pineapple**

1 Cup **Organic Spinach**

1/4 Cup **Organic Parsley**

1 tsp **Matcha Powder**

1 Tbsp **Chia Seeds**

1/2 tsp **Manuka Honey**

Fresh banana and berries, for serving

Green is the new gorgeous! This smoothie is not only high in antioxidants but also helps repair skin cells and boost collagen production to keep skin firm, toned, and glowing.

Instructions:

1. Place ingredients in a blender and purée until smooth and creamy.

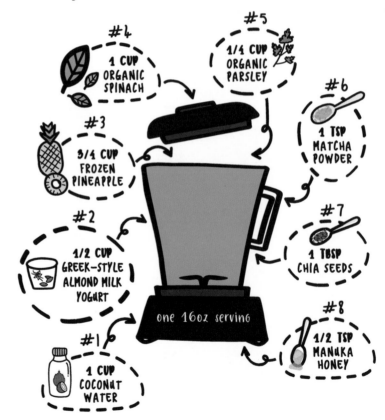

#4 1 CUP ORGANIC SPINACH

#5 1/4 CUP ORGANIC PARSLEY

#6 1 TSP MATCHA POWDER

#3 3/4 CUP FROZEN PINEAPPLE

#7 1 TBSP CHIA SEEDS

#2 1/2 CUP GREEK-STYLE ALMOND MILK YOGURT

one 16oz serving

#8 1/2 TSP MANUKA HONEY

#1 1 CUP COCONUT WATER

2. Pour into glass, garnish with fresh banana and berries, and serve immediately.

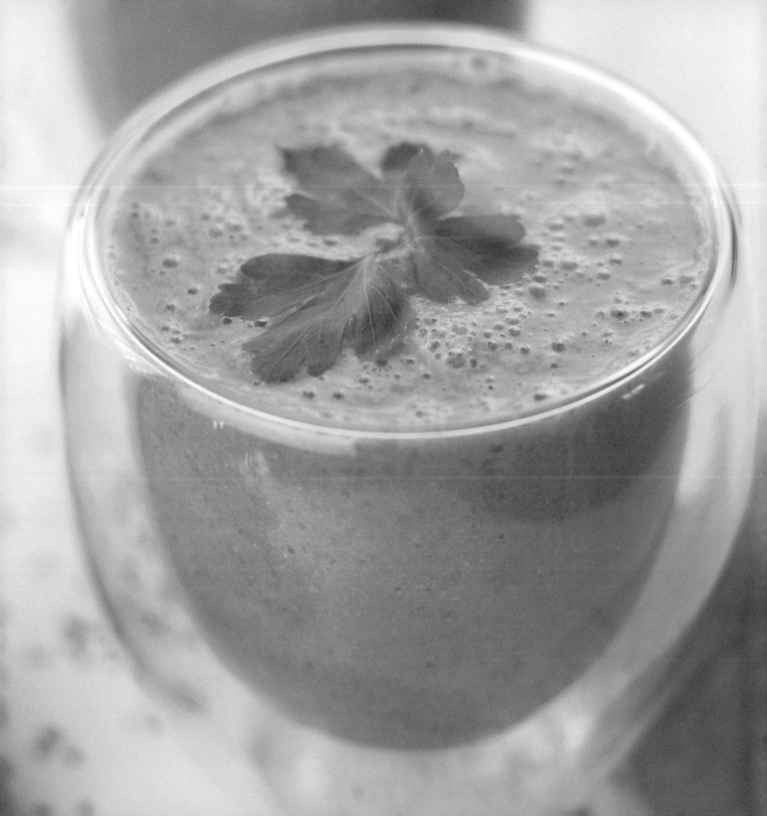

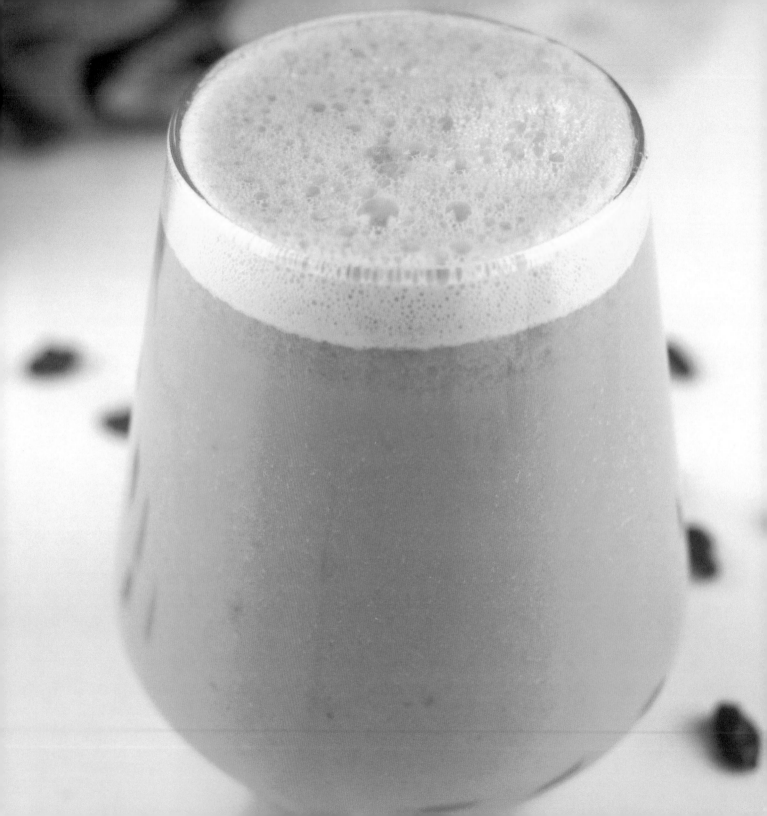

Kale Boost

This green smoothie, filled to the brim with antioxidants, vitamin C, and fiber, is delicious and great for digestion.

Instructions:

1. Place ingredients in a blender and purée until it is smooth.

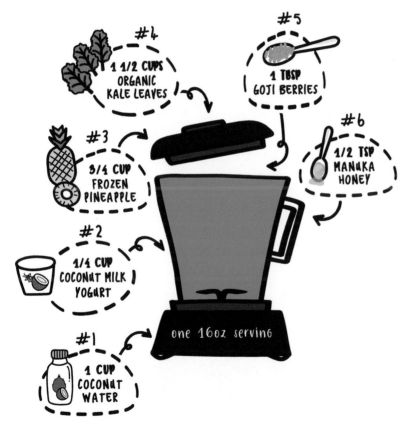

2. Pour into glass, garnish with goji berries, and serve immediately.

Ingredients:

1 Cup **Coconut Water**

1/4 Cup **Coconut Milk Yogurt (Plain or Vanilla Flavor)**

3/4 Cup **Frozen Pineapple**

1 1/2 Cups **Kale Leaves**

1 Tbsp **Goji Berries**

1/2 tsp **Manuka Honey**

Goji berries, for serving

Apple Green

With a bit of spice courtesy of its parsley component, this green smoothie is the perfect detoxifying treat.

Ingredients:

1 Cup **Apple Juice**

3/4 Cup **Frozen Pineapple**

1 Cup **Organic Green Apple Slices**

1 Cup **Organic Spinach**

1/4 Cup **Organic Parsley**

1 Tbsp **Chia Seeds**

1/2 tsp **Manuka Honey**

Fresh berries, for serving

Instructions:

1. Place ingredients in a blender and purée until smooth.

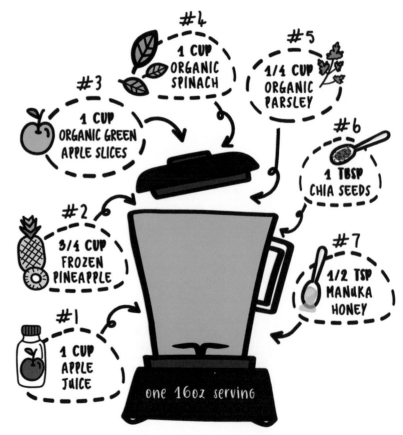

2. Pour into glass, garnish with some fresh berries, and serve immediately.

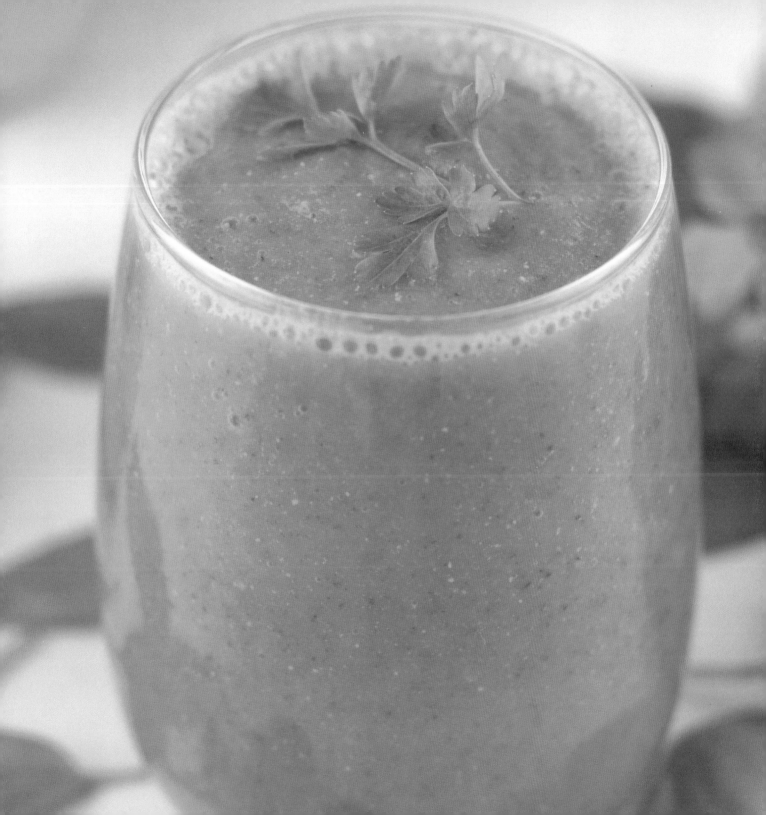

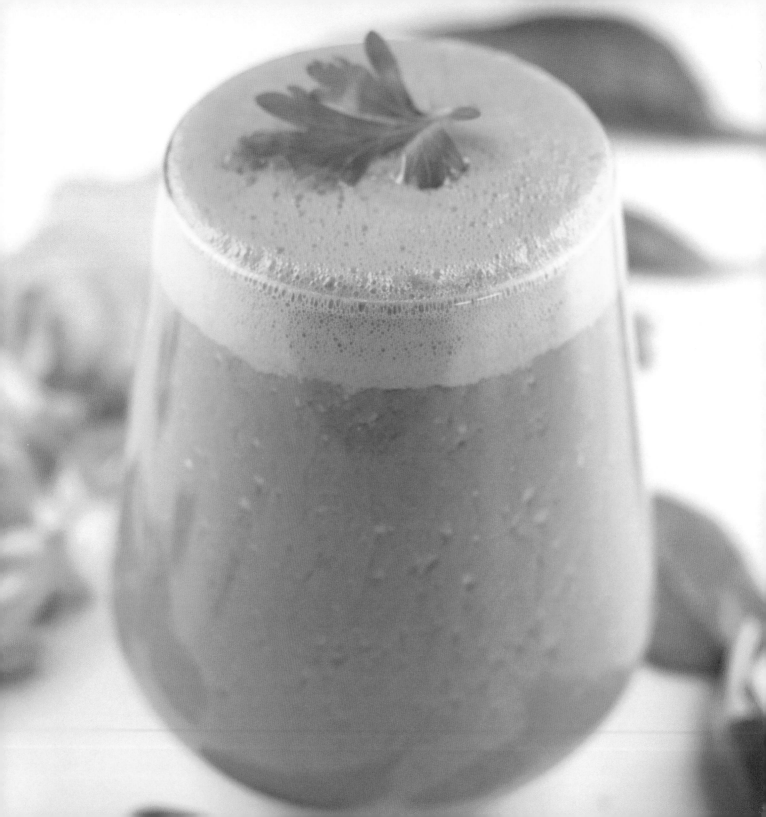

Parsley Green

This refreshing smoothie is packed with antioxidants and vitamin C, and great for immune boosting.

Instructions:

1. Place ingredients in a blender and purée until smooth.

Ingredients:

1 Cup **Coconut Water**

1/4 Cup **Coconut Milk Yogurt (Plain or Vanilla Flavor)**

3/4 Cup **Frozen Pineapple**

1 Cup **Organic Spinach**

1/4 Cup **Organic Parsley**

1 Tbsp **Sliced Fresh Ginger**

1/2 tsp **Manuka Honey**

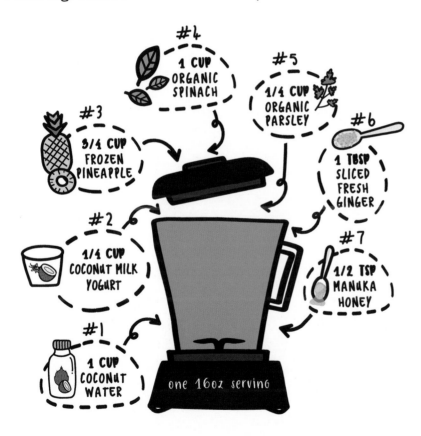

#4 1 CUP ORGANIC SPINACH

#5 1/4 CUP ORGANIC PARSLEY

#3 3/4 CUP FROZEN PINEAPPLE

#6 1 TBSP SLICED FRESH GINGER

#2 1/4 CUP COCONUT MILK YOGURT

#7 1/2 TSP MANUKA HONEY

#1 1 CUP COCONUT WATER

one 16oz serving

2. Pour into glass and serve immediately.

HIGH ANTIOXIDANTS

39

SuperGreen

Ingredients:

1 Cup **Coconut Water**

1/4 Cup **Coconut Milk Yogurt (Plain or Vanilla Flavor)**

3/4 Cup **Frozen Pineapple**

1 Cup **Organic Kale Leaves**

3/4 Cup **Organic Spinach**

7 **Mint Leaves**

1 Tbsp **Chia Seeds**

1/2 tsp **Manuka Honey**

With three different kinds of greens--kale, spinach, and mint--this drink lives up to its name and packs a superfood punch of nutrients and antioxidants.

Instructions:

1. Place ingredients in a blender and purée until smooth and creamy.

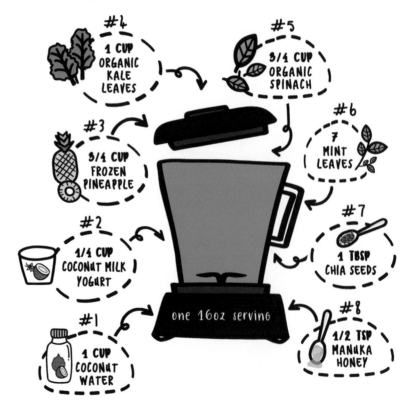

2. Pour into glass, garnish with fresh berries, and serve immediately.

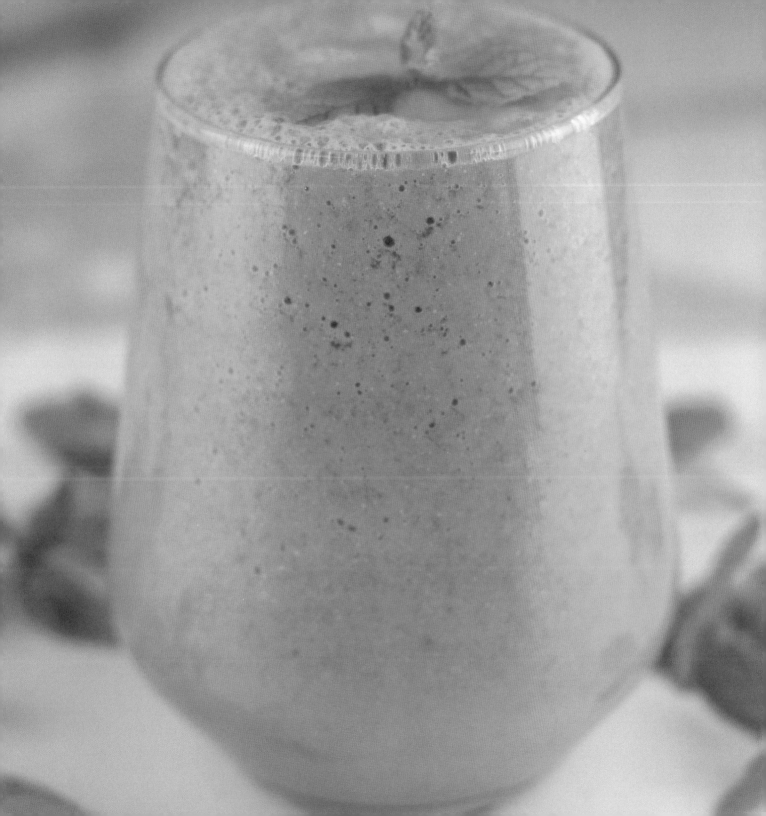

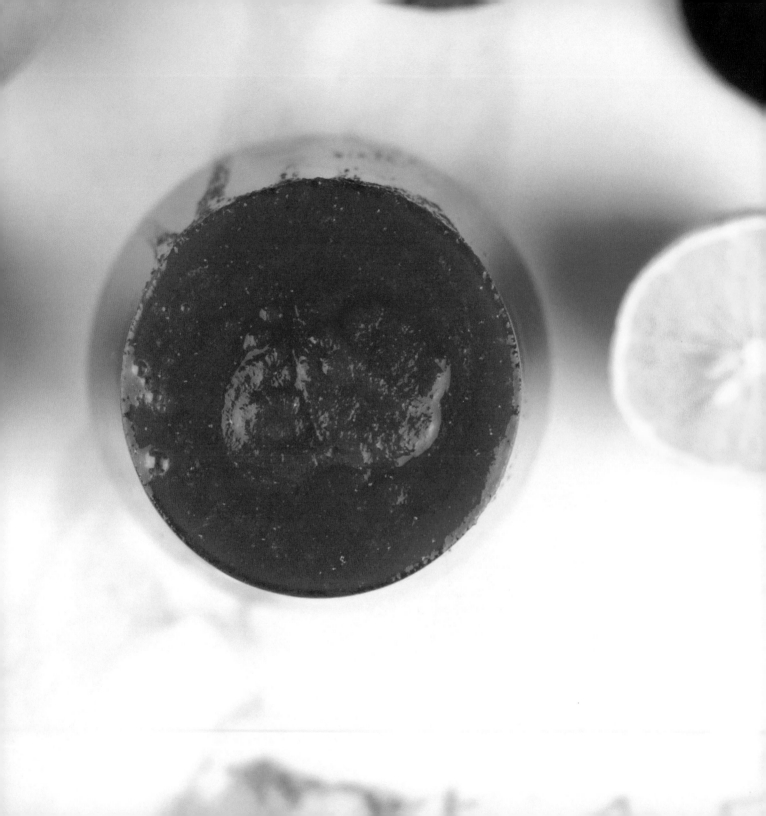

Chapter 3:
Detox & Cleanse

Turmeric Mango

Ingredients:

1 1/4 Cups **Coconut Water**

1/4 Cup **Coconut Milk Yogurt (Plain or Vanilla Flavor)**

1/2 Cup **Frozen Pineapple**

1 Cup **Frozen Mangoes**

1/2 Cup **Shredded Carrots**

1/2 tsp **Turmeric Powder**

1/2 tsp **Manuka Honey**

Loaded with Vitamin C, this detoxing smoothie not only helps remove toxins but also anti-inflammatory.

Instructions:

1. Place ingredients in a blender and purée until it is smooth.

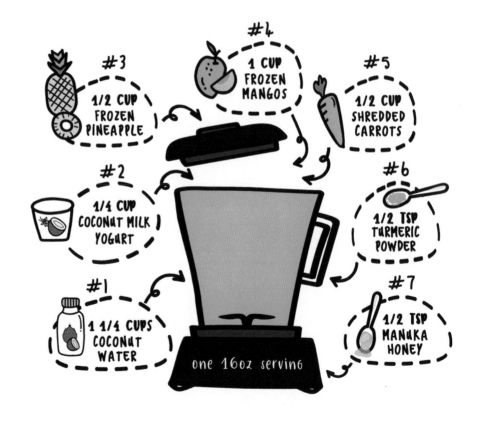

#3 1/2 CUP FROZEN PINEAPPLE

#4 1 CUP FROZEN MANGOS

#5 1/2 CUP SHREDDED CARROTS

#2 1/4 CUP COCONUT MILK YOGURT

#6 1/2 TSP TURMERIC POWDER

#1 1 1/4 CUPS COCONUT WATER

#7 1/2 TSP MANUKA HONEY

one 16oz serving

2. Pour into glass and serve immediately.

DETOXIFYING

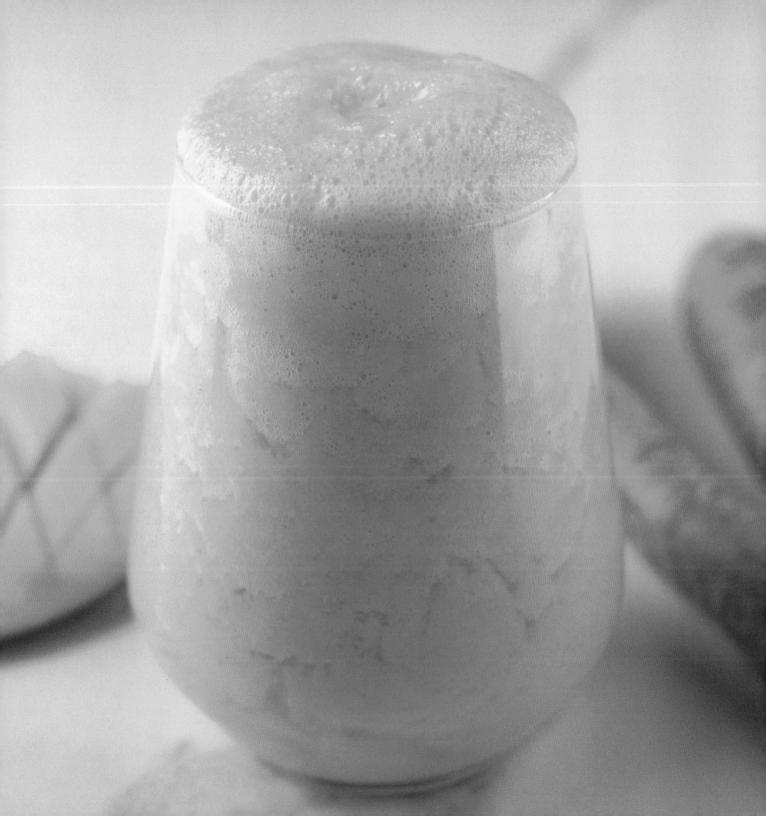

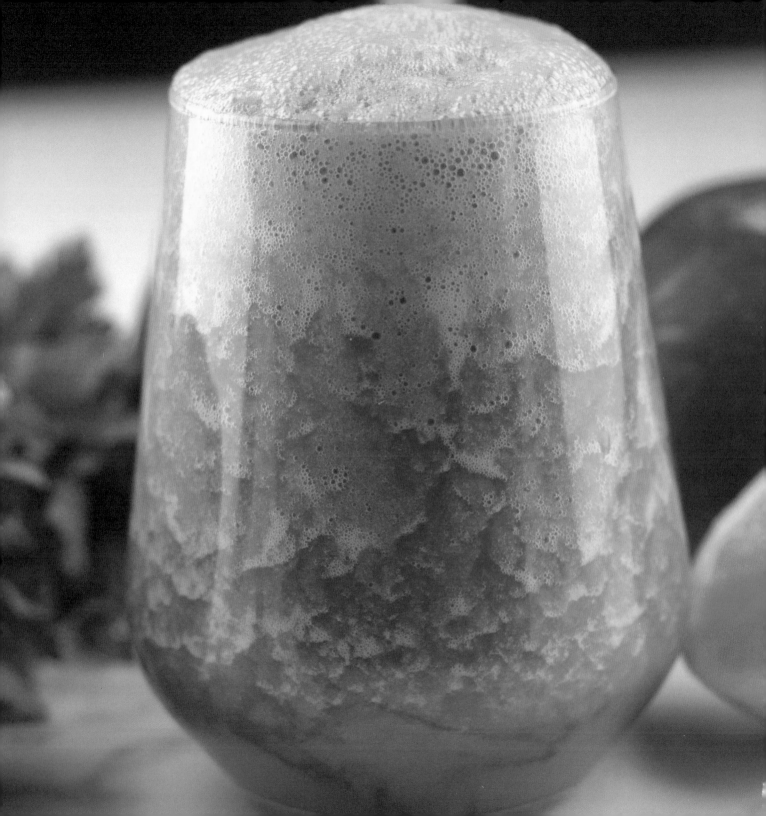

Turmeric Cilantro

This refreshing smoothie is loaded with antioxidants and nutrients. It is great for boosting the immune system and cleansing the kidneys.

Instructions:

1. Place ingredients in a blender and purée until smooth.

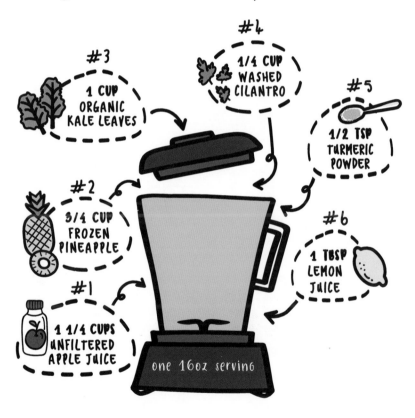

#3 1 CUP ORGANIC KALE LEAVES

#4 1/4 CUP WASHED CILANTRO

#5 1/2 TSP TURMERIC POWDER

#2 3/4 CUP FROZEN PINEAPPLE

#6 1 TBSP LEMON JUICE

#1 1 1/4 CUPS UNFILTERED APPLE JUICE

one 16oz serving

2. Pour into glass, sprinkle with some ground black pepper, and serve immediately.

Ingredients:

1 1/4 Cups **Apple Juice**

3/4 Cup **Frozen Pineapple**

1 Cup **Organic Kale Leaves**

1/4 Cup **Organic Cilantro**

1/2 tsp **Turmeric Powder**

1 Tbsp **Fresh Lemon Juice**

A Few Sprinkles **Ground Black Pepper**

DETOXIFYING

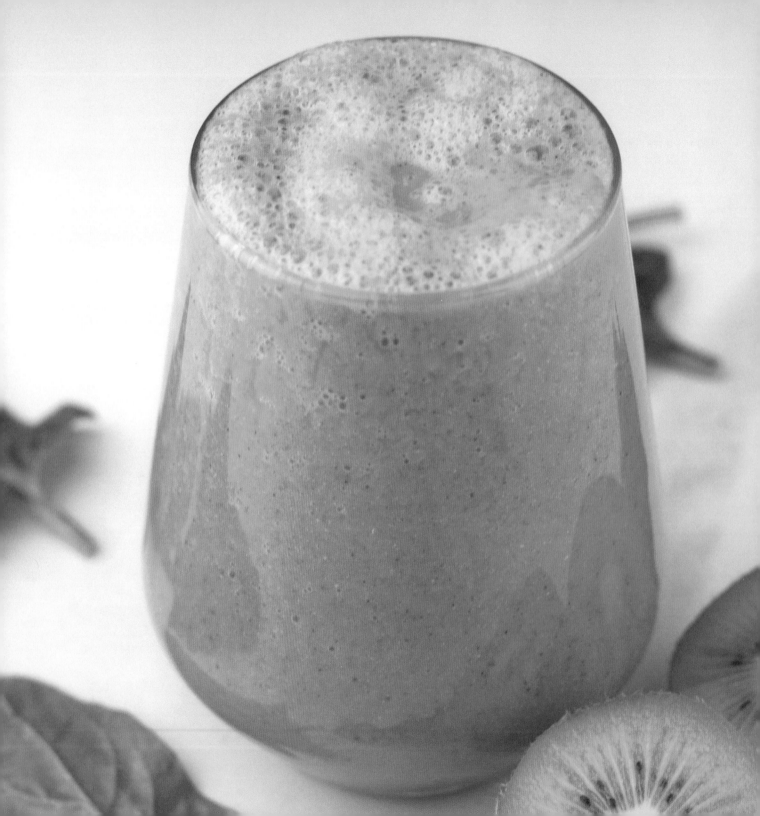

Kiwi Boost

Loaded with antioxidants and vitamin C, this detoxing smoothie helps boost immunity and collagen production.

Instructions:

1. Place ingredients in a blender and purée until it is smooth.

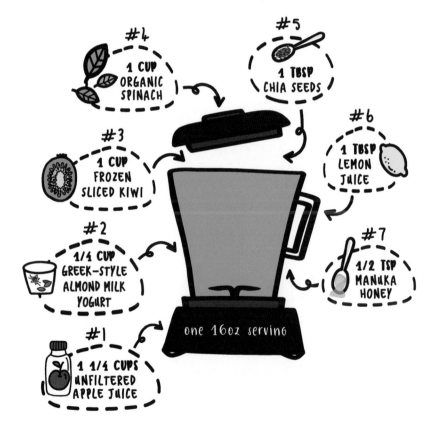

#4 1 CUP ORGANIC SPINACH

#5 1 TBSP CHIA SEEDS

#3 1 CUP FROZEN SLICED KIWI

#6 1 TBSP LEMON JUICE

#2 1/4 CUP GREEK-STYLE ALMOND MILK YOGURT

#7 1/2 TSP MANUKA HONEY

#1 1 1/4 CUPS UNFILTERED APPLE JUICE

one 16oz serving

2. Pour into glass, garnish with fresh berries or pomegranate seeds, and serve immediately.

Ingredients:

1 1/4 Cups **Apple Juice**

1/4 Cup **Greek-Style Almond Milk Yogurt (Plain or Vanilla Flavor)**

1 Cup **Frozen Sliced Kiwi**

1 Cup **Organic Spinach**

1 Tbsp **Chia Seeds**

1 Tbsp **Fresh Lemon Juice**

1/2 tsp **Manuka Honey**

Fresh berries or pomegranate seeds, for serving

HIGH VITAMIN C

Beet Apple Carrot

Loaded with nutrients, this detoxing smoothie not only helps remove toxins from liver but also ant- inflammatory.

Ingredients:

1 1/4 Cups **Filtered Water**

3/4 Cup **Steamed Beet Root**

1 Cup **Organic Green Apple Slices**

1/2 Cup **ShreddedCarrots**

1 Tbsp **Chia Seeds**

1 Tbsp **Fresh Lemon Juice**

Instructions:

1. Place ingredients in a blender and purée until smooth.

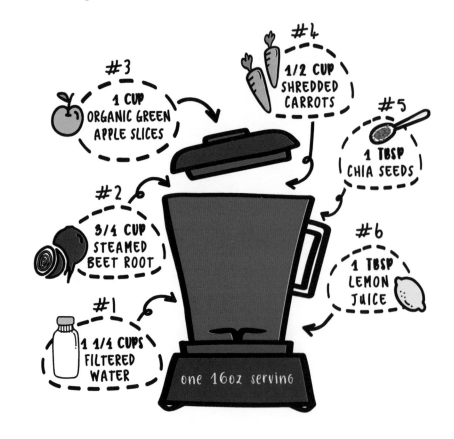

#3
1 CUP ORGANIC GREEN APPLE SLICES

#4
1/2 CUP SHREDDED CARROTS

#5
1 TBSP CHIA SEEDS

#2
3/4 CUP STEAMED BEET ROOT

#6
1 TBSP LEMON JUICE

#1
1 1/4 CUPS FILTERED WATER

one 16oz serving

2. Pour into glass and serve immediately.

DETOXIFYING

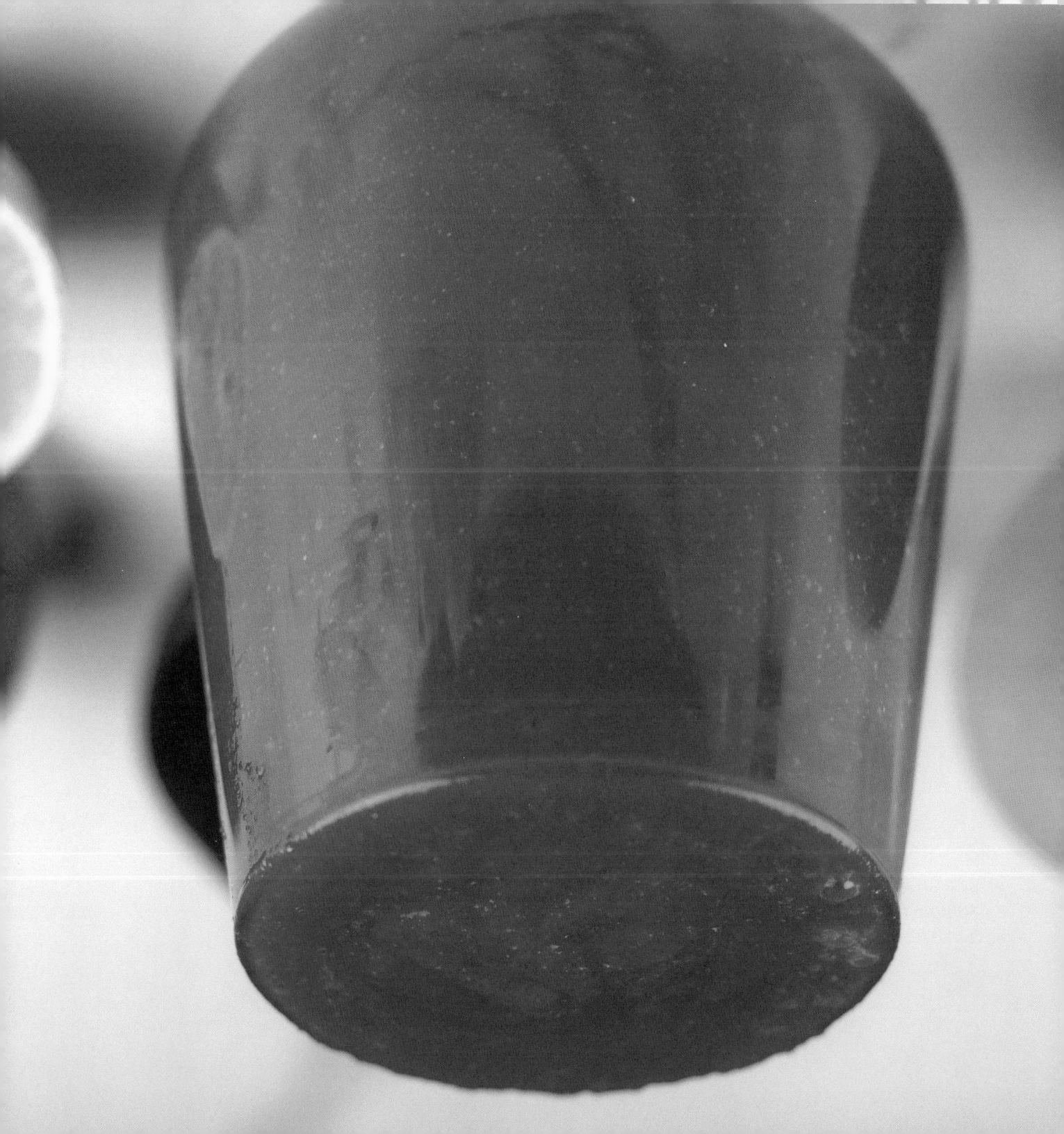

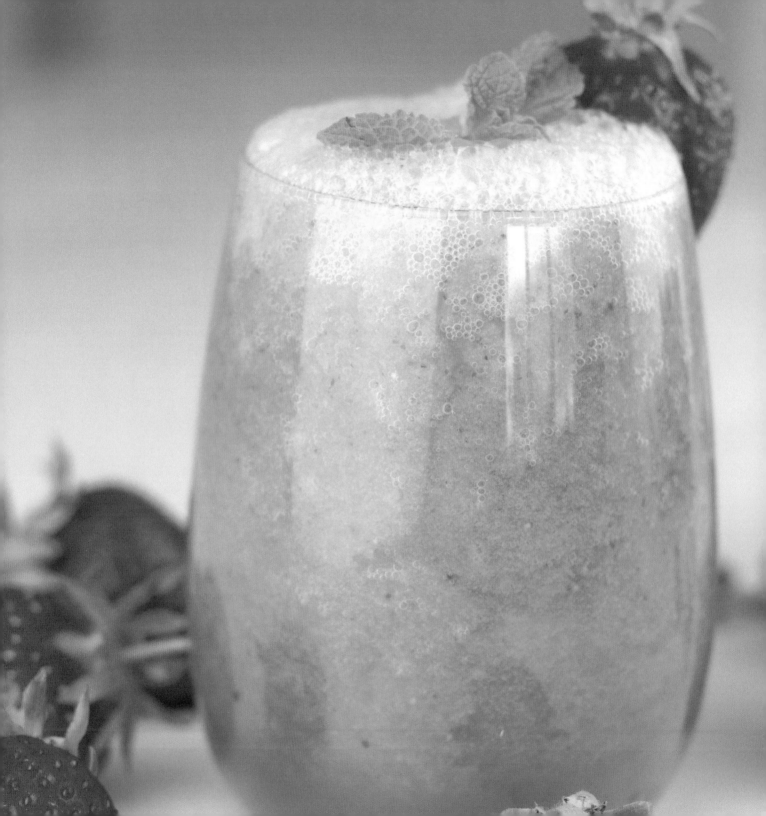

Spa Treat

Escape to the spa in your mind with this smoothie that's not just chock-full of vitamin C and antioxidants, but ultra-hydrating thanks to its coconut water, melon, and cucumber. You'll feel renewed after just a few sips.

Instructions:

1. Place ingredients in a blender and purée until smooth.

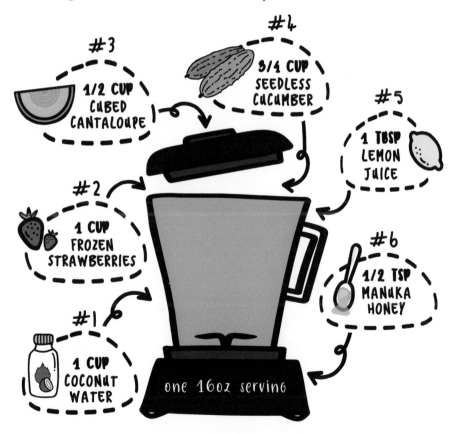

2. Pour into glass and serve immediately.

Cranberry Cleansing

Ingredients:

1 Cup **Unsweetened Cranberry Juice**

1 Cup **Frozen Cranberrries**

3/4 Cup **Orange Slices**

1/4 Cup **Red Seedless Grapes**

1 Tbsp **Fresh Lemon Juice**

1/2 tsp **Manuka Honey**

A cranberry juice base gives this smoothie the distinct ability to remove toxins from the liver and kidneys--a perfect antidote when you've had one too many drinks.

Instructions:

1. Place ingredients in a blender and purée until smooth.

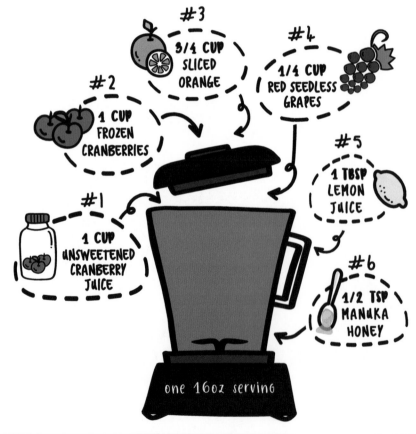

#2 1 CUP FROZEN CRANBERRIES

#3 3/4 CUP SLICED ORANGE

#4 1/4 CUP RED SEEDLESS GRAPES

#5 1 TBSP LEMON JUICE

#1 1 CUP UNSWEETENED CRANBERRY JUICE

#6 1/2 TSP MANUKA HONEY

one 16oz serving

2. Pour into glass and serve immediately.

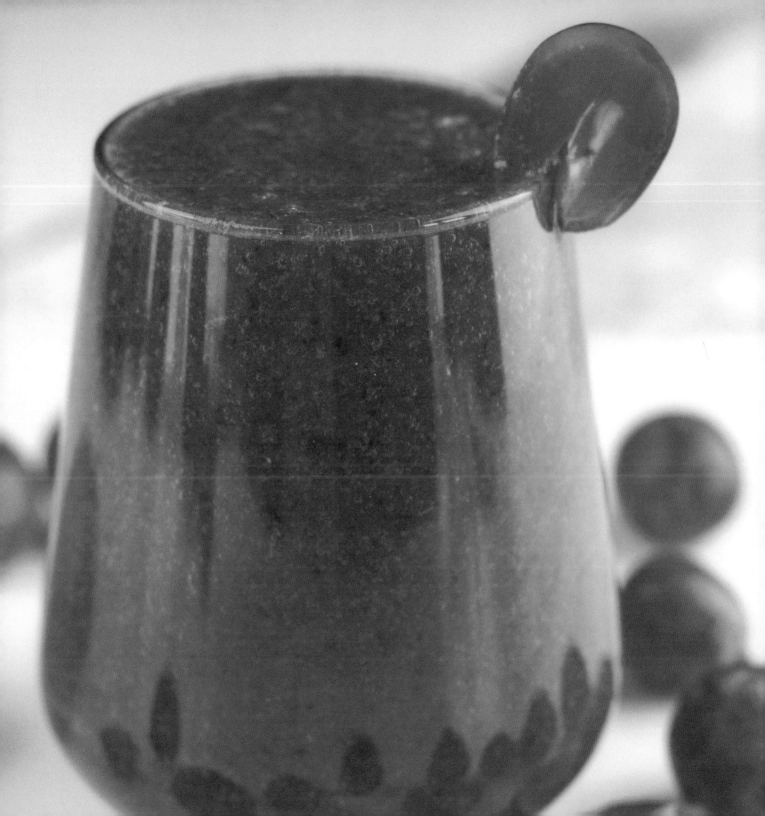

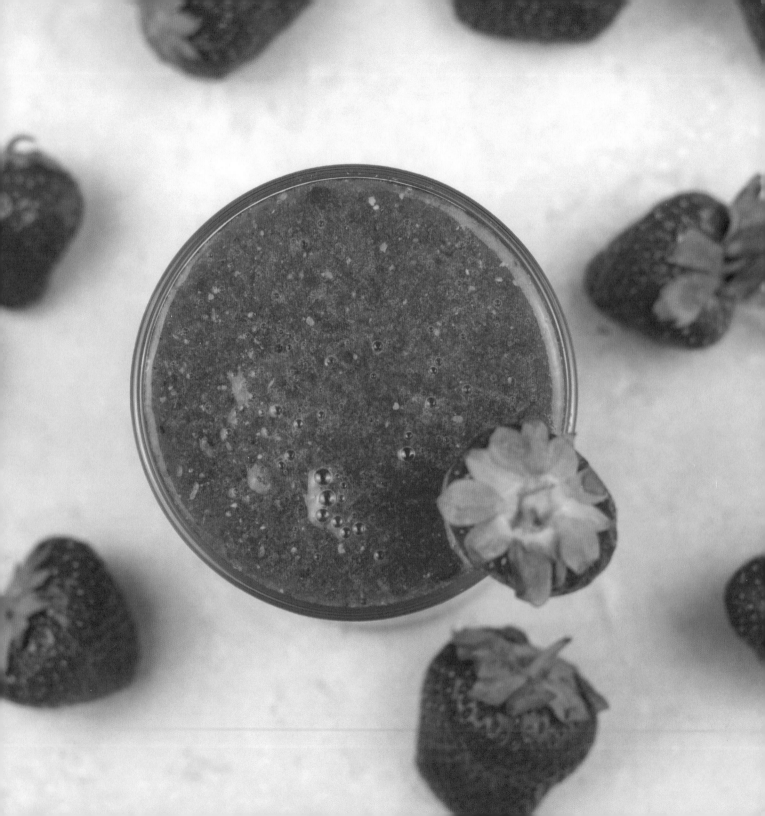

Chapter 4:

Immune Boosters

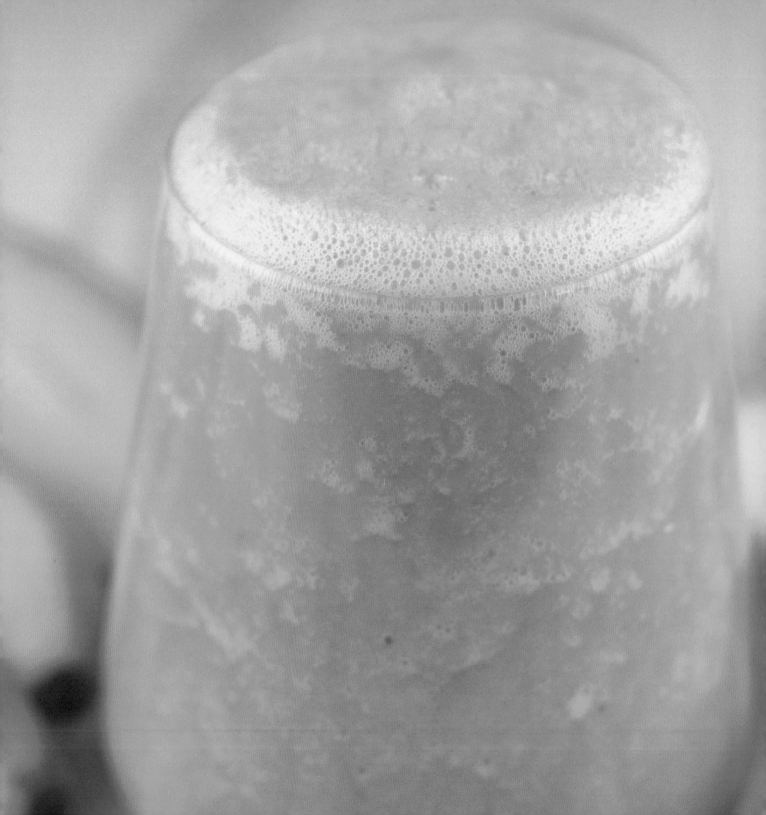

Citrus Boost

This gorgeous orange smoothie provides all the vitamin C and antioxidants needed to prevent a cold.

Instructions:

1. Place ingredients in a blender and purée until smooth.

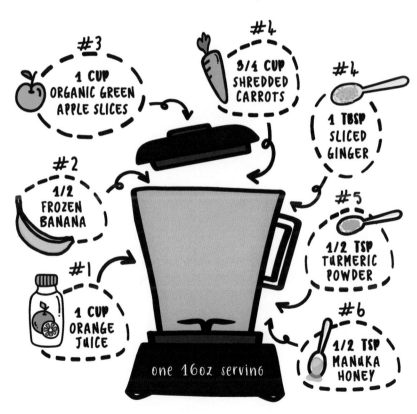

#3
1 CUP ORGANIC GREEN APPLE SLICES

#4
3/4 CUP SHREDDED CARROTS

#4
1 TBSP SLICED GINGER

#2
1/2 FROZEN BANANA

#5
1/2 TSP TURMERIC POWDER

#1
1 CUP ORANGE JUICE

#6
1/2 TSP MANUKA HONEY

one 16oz serving

2. Pour into glass and serve immediately.

Ingredients:

1 Cup **Orange Juice**
1/2 **Froze Banana**
1 Cup **Organic Green Apple Slices**
3/4 Cup **Shredded Carrots**
1 Tbsp **Sliced Fresh Ginger**
1/2 tsp **Turmeric Powder**
1/2 tsp **Manuka Honey**

HIGH VITAMIN C

Carrot Cooler

Ingredients:

1 Cup **Orange Juice**

1/4 Cup **Coconut Milk Yogurt (Plain or Vanilla Flavor)**

3/4 Cup **Frozen Pineapple**

3/4 Cup **Shredded Carrots**

1 Tbsp **Sliced Fresh Ginger**

1 Tbsp **Hemp Hearts**

1/2 tsp **Manuka Honey**

Loaded with beta-carotene and vitamin C, this nutrient-dense smoothie is great for eyes, skin, and digestion.

Instructions:

1. Place ingredients in a blender and purée until smooth.

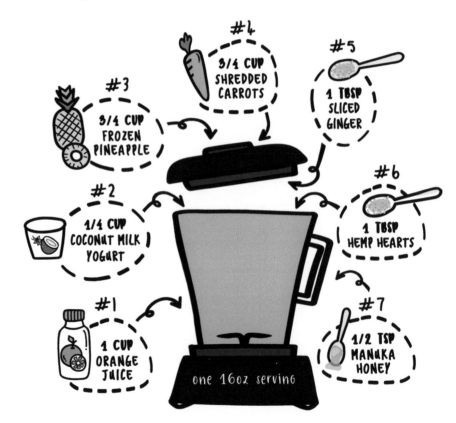

2. Pour into glass and serve immediately.

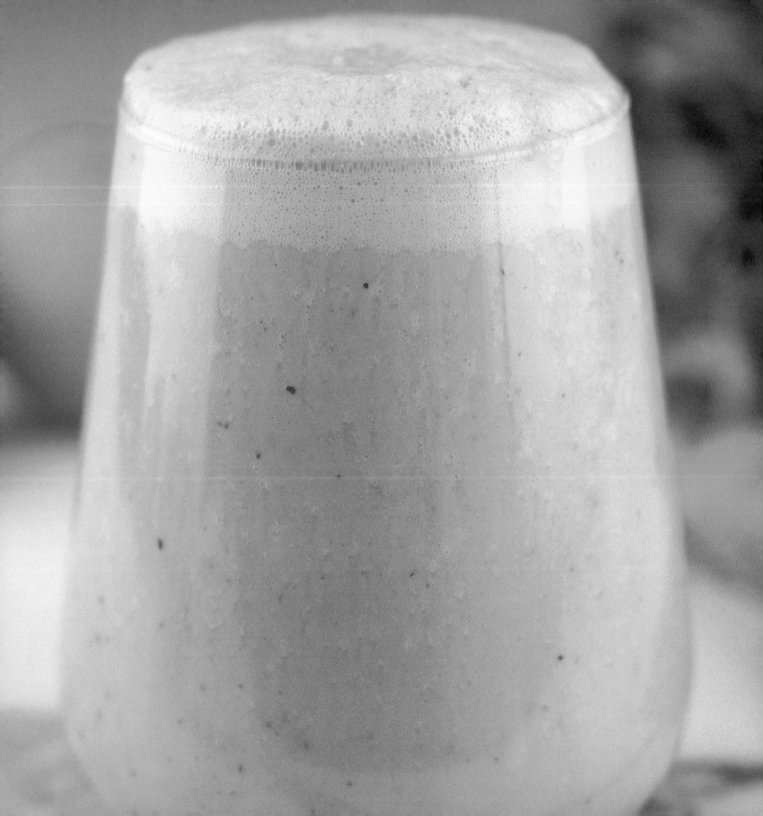

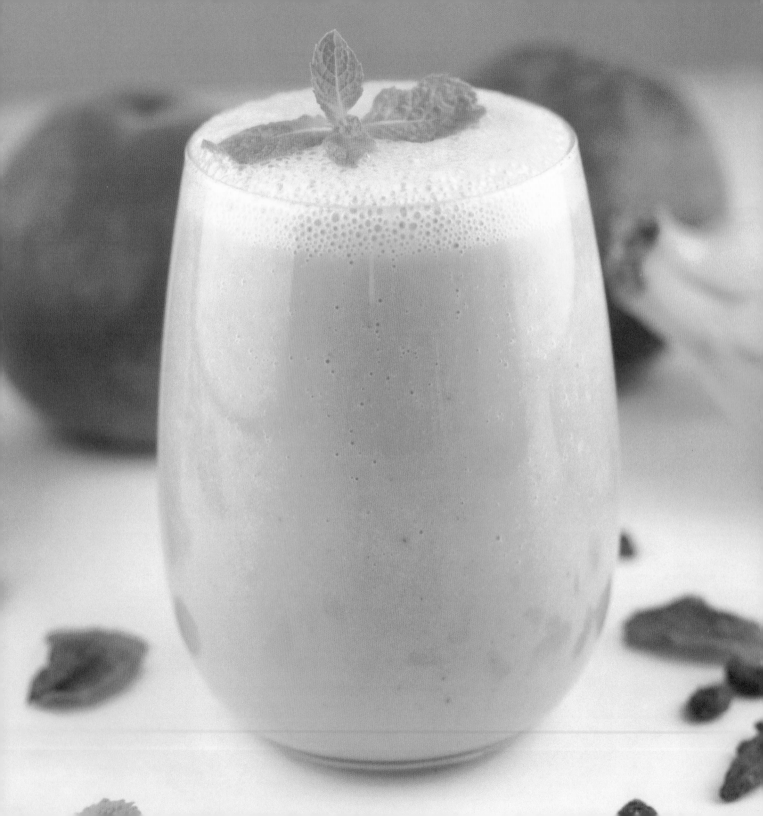

Peach & Ginger

Spiced with ginger, this peachy and immunity-boosting smoothie is loaded with antioxidants, fiber, and vitamin C.

Instructions:

1. Place ingredients in a blender and purée until smooth.

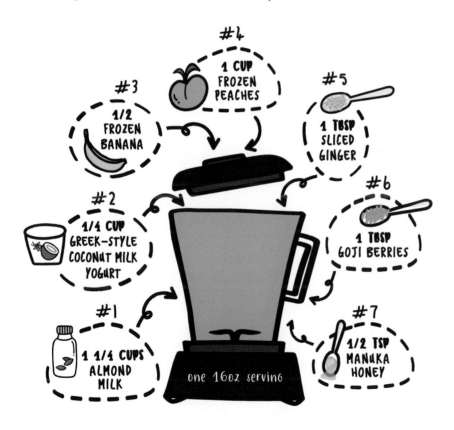

2. Pour into glass and serve immediately.

Ingredients:

1 1/4 Cup **Almond Milk**

1/4 Cup **Greek-Style Coconut Milk Yogurt (Plain or Vanilla Flavor)**

1/2 **Frozen Banana**

1 Cup **Frozen Peaches**

1 Tbsp **Sliced Fresh Ginger**

1 Tbsp **Goji Berries**

1/2 tsp **Manuka Honey**

HIGH FIBER

Strawberry Lemonade

Ingredients:

1/4 Cup **Fresh Lemon Juice**
1 1/2 Cups **Filtered Water**
1 1/2 Cups **Frozen Strawberries**
1 Tbsp **Goji Berries**
1 Tbsp **Chia Seeds**
1 tsp **Manuka Honey**

Loaded with vitamin C and nutrients, this immunity-boosting smoothie tastes just like summer in a cup!

Instructions:

1. Place ingredients in a blender and purée until smooth.

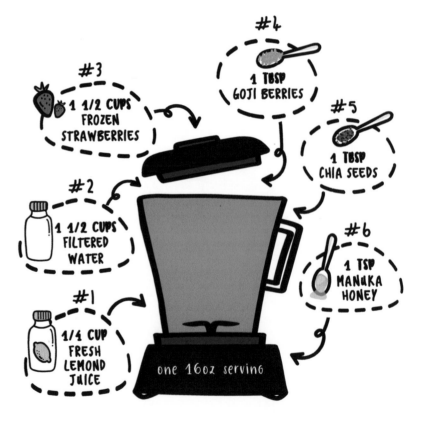

#3 1 1/2 CUPS FROZEN STRAWBERRIES

#4 1 TBSP GOJI BERRIES

#5 1 TBSP CHIA SEEDS

#2 1 1/2 CUPS FILTERED WATER

#6 1 TSP MANUKA HONEY

#1 1/4 CUP FRESH LEMOND JUICE

one 16oz serving

2. Pour into glass and serve immediately.

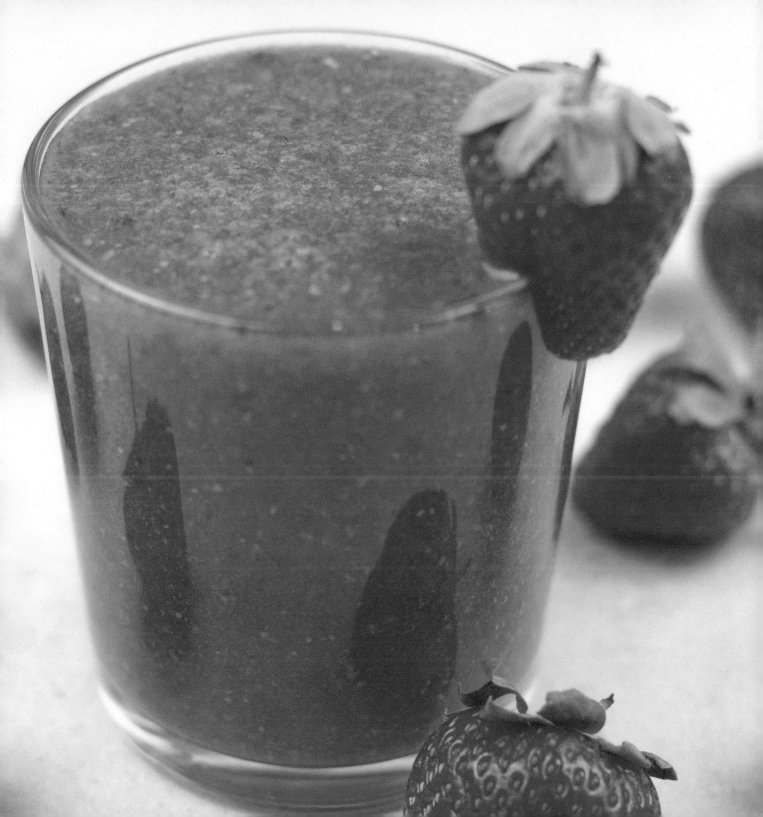

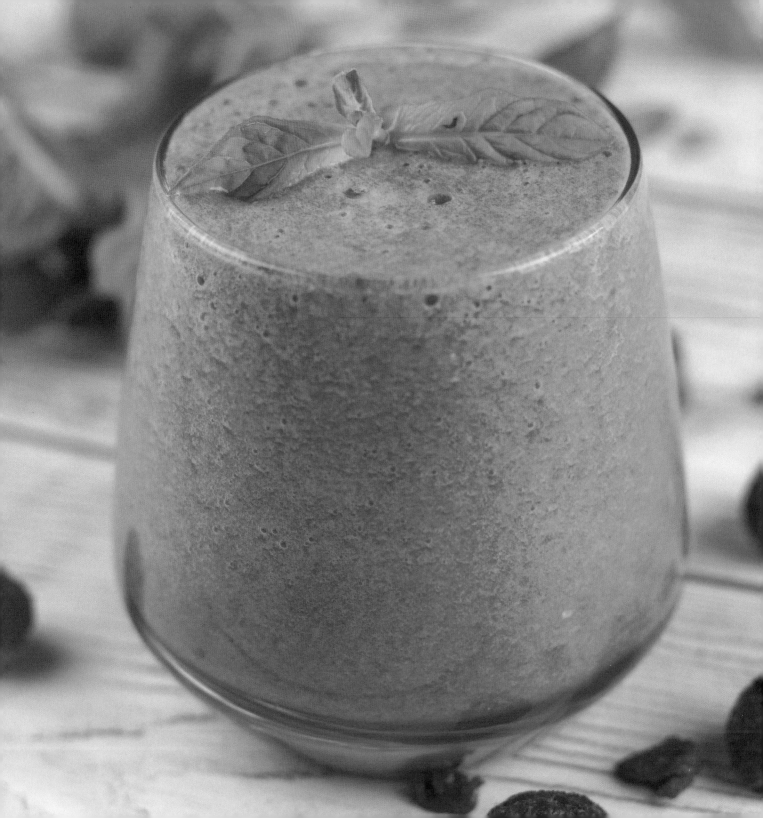

Raspberry Boost

This immune-boosting, ruby-red drink is deliciously sweet. Pineapple, hemp hearts and manuka honey give it the benefit of being good for digestion, hair, skin, nails, and immunity.

Instructions:

1. Place ingredients in a blender and purée until smooth.

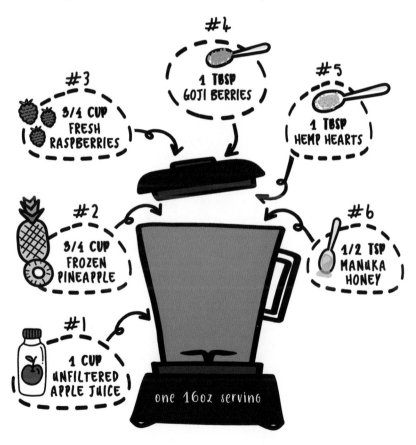

2. Pour into glass and serve immediately.

Ingredients:

1 Cup **Unfiltered Apple Juice**
3/4 Cup **Frozen Pineapple**
3/4 Cup **Fresh Raspberries**
1 Tbsp **Goji Berries**
1 Tbsp **Hemp Hearts**
1/2 tsp **Manuka Honey**

HIGH ANTIOXIDANTS

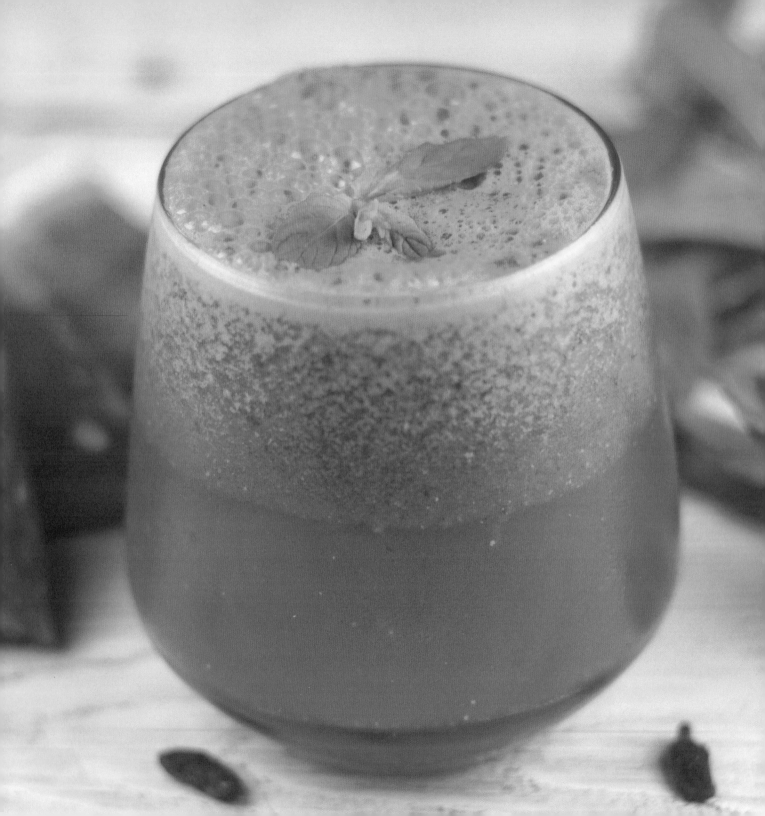

Watermelon Boost

With minty flavor, this refreshing smoothie is also filled to the brim with cancer-fighting omega-3 fatty acids thanks to its watermelon and antioxidants from the added goji berries.

Instructions:

1. Place ingredients in a blender and purée until smooth.

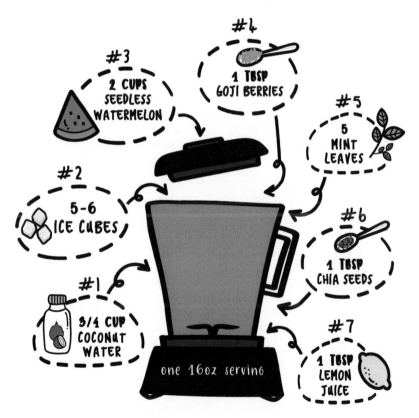

2. Pour into glass and serve immediately.

Ingredients:

3/4 Cup **Coconut Water**

5-6 **Ice Cubes**

2 Cups **Seedless Watermelon**

1 Tbsp **Goji Berries**

5 of **Mint Leaves**

1 Tbsp **Chia Seeds**

1 Tbsp **Fresh Lemon Juice**

HIGH ANTIOXIDANTS

69

Blueberry Boost

Ingredients:

1 1/4 Cups **Almond Milk**

1/4 Cup **Greek-Style Coconut Milk Yogurt (Plain or Vanilla Flavor)**

1 Cup **Frozen Blueberries**

1/2 **Avocado**

1 Tbsp **Sliced Fresh Ginger**

1/2 tsp **Manuka Honey**

With a hint of spice from its fresh ginger, this fiberful, heart-healthy smoothie is a great morning kickstarter.

Instructions:

1. Place ingredients in a blender and purée until smooth.

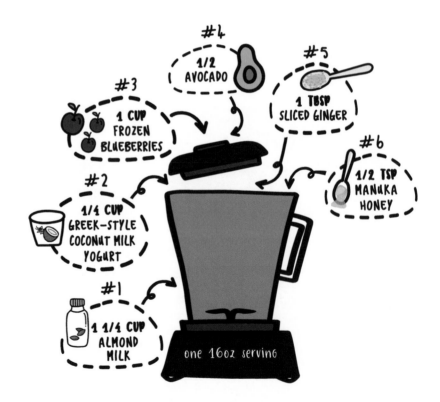

2. Pour into glass and serve immediately.

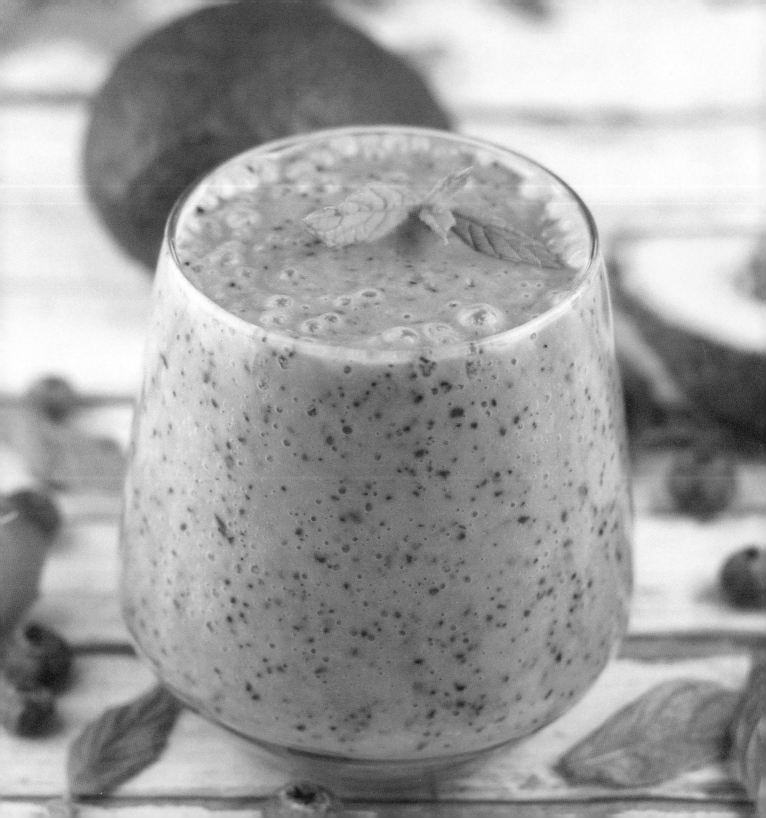

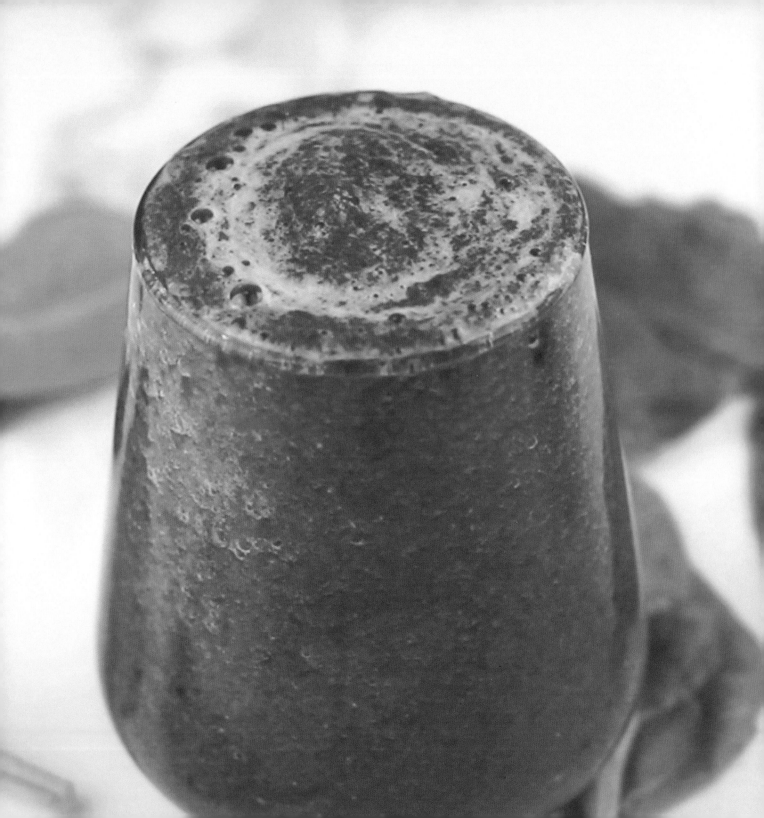

Blackberry Green

This immunity-boosting smoothie is not only refreshing but also loaded with antioxidants, nutrients, and vitamin C.

Instructions:

1. Place ingredients in a blender and purée until smooth.

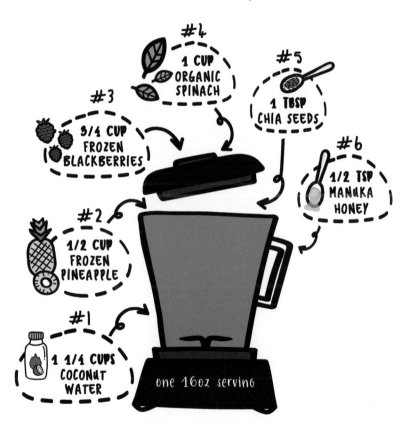

#4 1 CUP ORGANIC SPINACH

#5 1 TBSP CHIA SEEDS

#3 3/4 CUP FROZEN BLACKBERRIES

#6 1/2 TSP MANUKA HONEY

#2 1/2 CUP FROZEN PINEAPPLE

#1 1 1/4 CUPS COCONUT WATER

one 16oz serving

2. Pour into glass and serve immediately.

Ingredients:

1 1/4 Cups **Coconut Water**

1/2 Cup **Frozen Pineapple**

3/4 Cup **Organic Blackberries**

1 Cup **Organic Spinach**

1 Tbsp **Chai Seeds**

1/2 tsp **Manuka Honey**

HIGH ANTIOXIDANTS

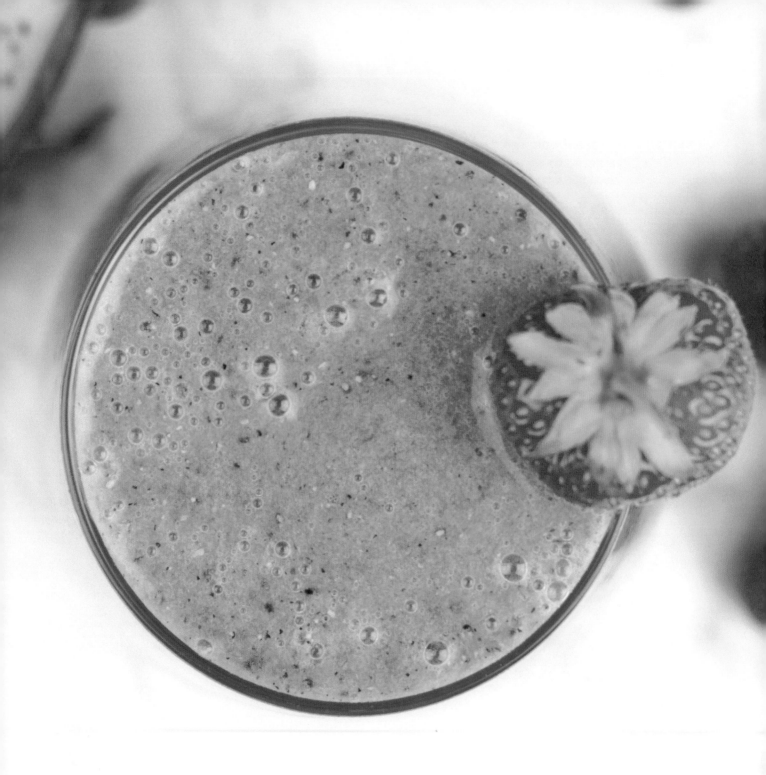

Chapter 5:

Tropical fruits

Lychee Boost

Ingredients:

1 Cup **Coconut Water**

1/4 Cup **Greek-Style Coconut Milk Yogurt (Plain or Vanilla Flavor)**

4-5 **Ice Cubes**

3/4 Cup **Seedless Lychee**

1 tsp **Vanilla Extract**

This refreshing smoothie is great for any party or just as self indulgent treat.

Instructions:

1. Place ingredients in a blender and purée until smooth.

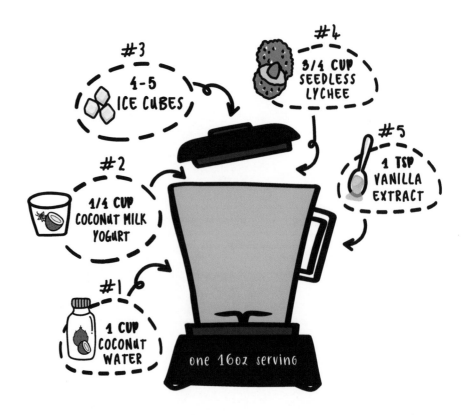

#3
4-5
ICE CUBES

#4
3/4 CUP
SEEDLESS
LYCHEE

#5
1 TSP
VANILLA
EXTRACT

#2
1/4 CUP
COCONUT MILK
YOGURT

#1
1 CUP
COCONUT
WATER

one 16oz serving

2. Pour into glass and serve immediately.

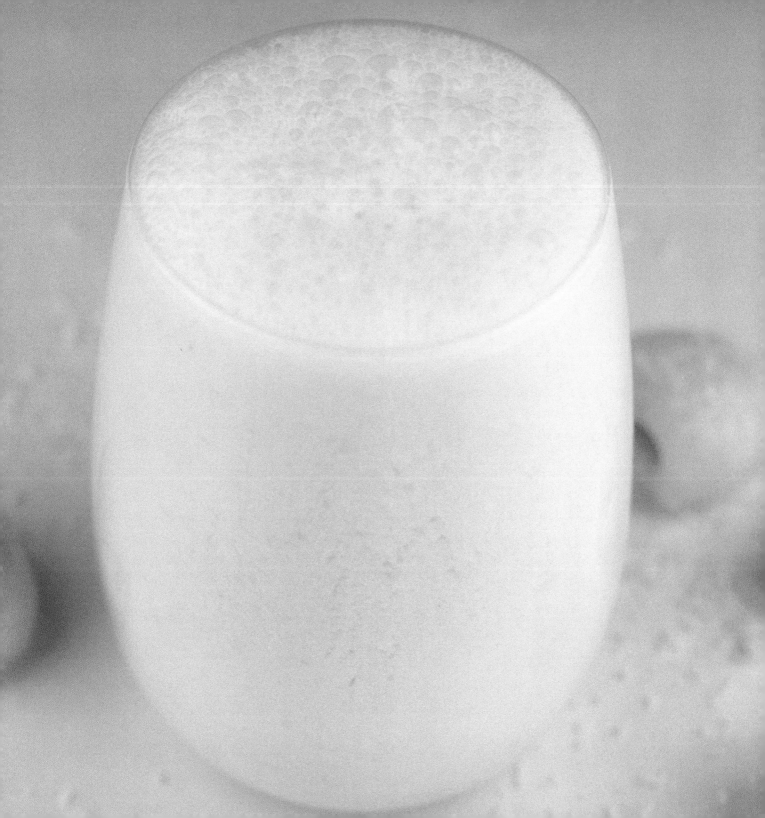

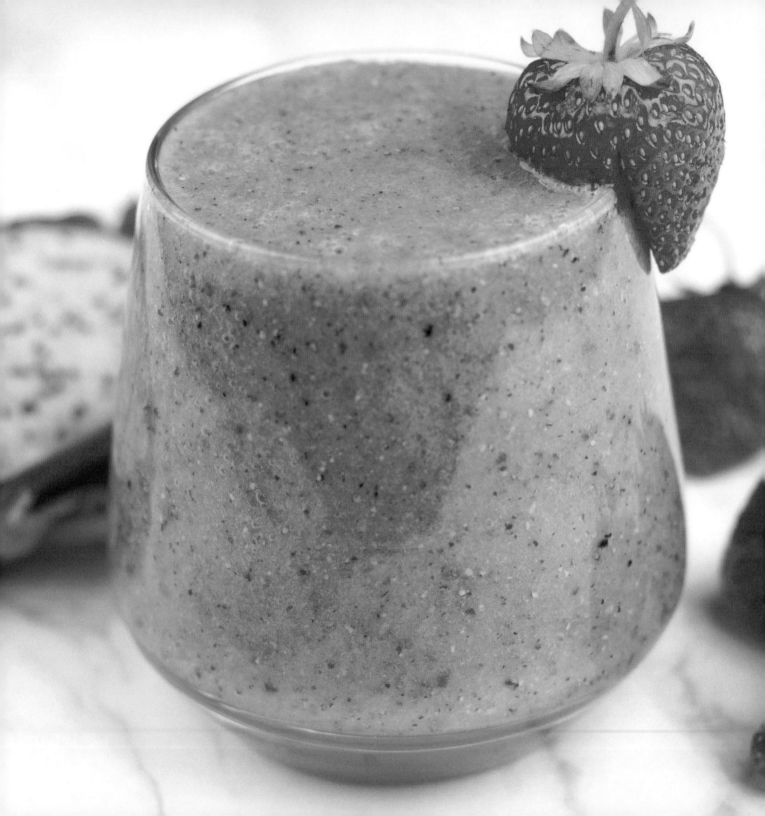

Pitaya Boost

This exotic fruit -- Pitaya (sometimes called dragon fruit) -- smoothie is jam-packed with antioxidants, nutrients, fiber, prebiotics, and vitamin C.

Instructions:

1. Place ingredients in a blender and purée until it is smooth.

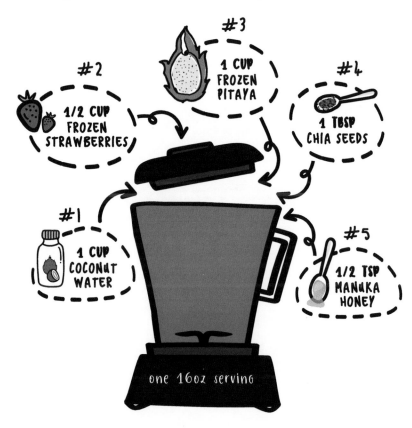

2. Pour into glass and serve immediately.

Ingredients:

1 Cup **Coconut Water**

1/2 Cup **Frozen Strawberries**

1 Cup **Frozen Pitaya**

1 Tbsp **Chia Seeds**

1/2 tsp **Manuka Honey**

HIGH VITAMIN C

Coconut Colada

Ingredients:

1 Cup **Pineapple Juice**

1/2 Cup **Greek-Style Coconut Milk Yogurt (Plain or Vanilla Flavor)**

3/4 Cup **Frozen Pineapple**

1/2 Cup **Coconut Meat**

1 Tbsp **Ground Flaxseed**

1/2 tsp **Manuka Honey**

Loaded with antioxidants, MCT, and fiber, this delicious tropical smoothie is great for a poolside delight or a drab day when you're dreaming of the sun.

Instructions:

1. Place ingredients in a blender and purée until smooth.

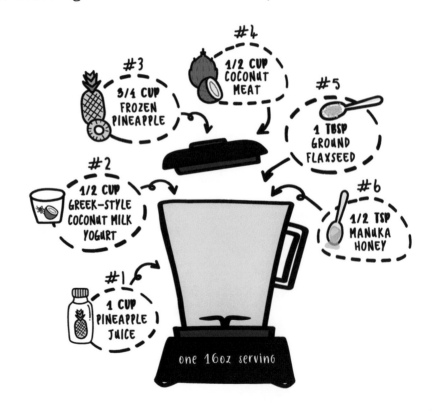

#4 1/2 CUP COCONUT MEAT

#3 3/4 CUP FROZEN PINEAPPLE

#5 1 TBSP GROUND FLAXSEED

#2 1/2 CUP GREEK-STYLE COCONUT MILK YOGURT

#6 1/2 TSP MANUKA HONEY

#1 1 CUP PINEAPPLE JUICE

one 16oz serving

2. Pour into glass and serve immediately.

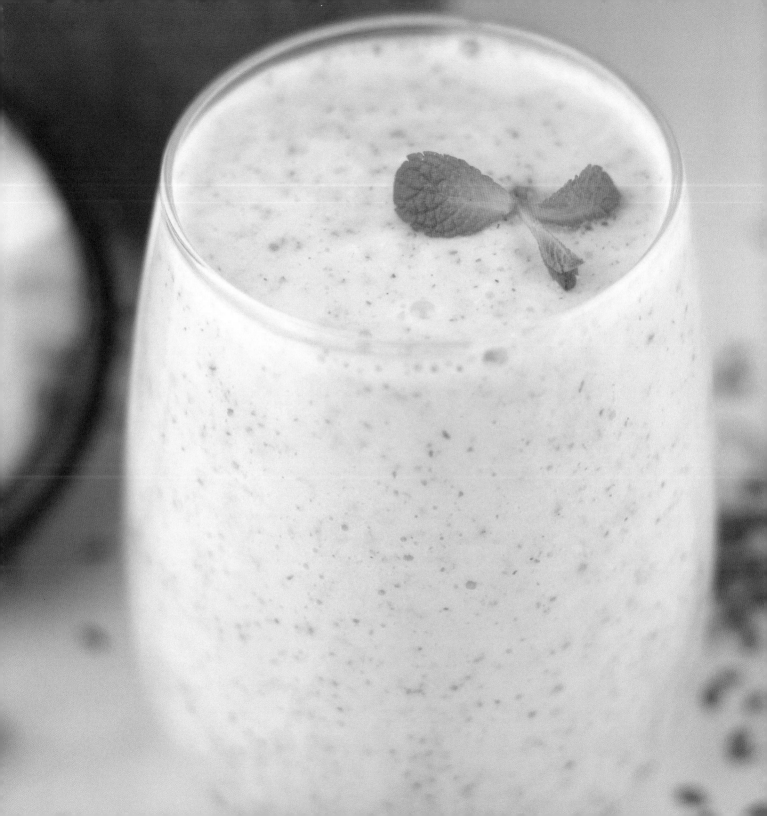

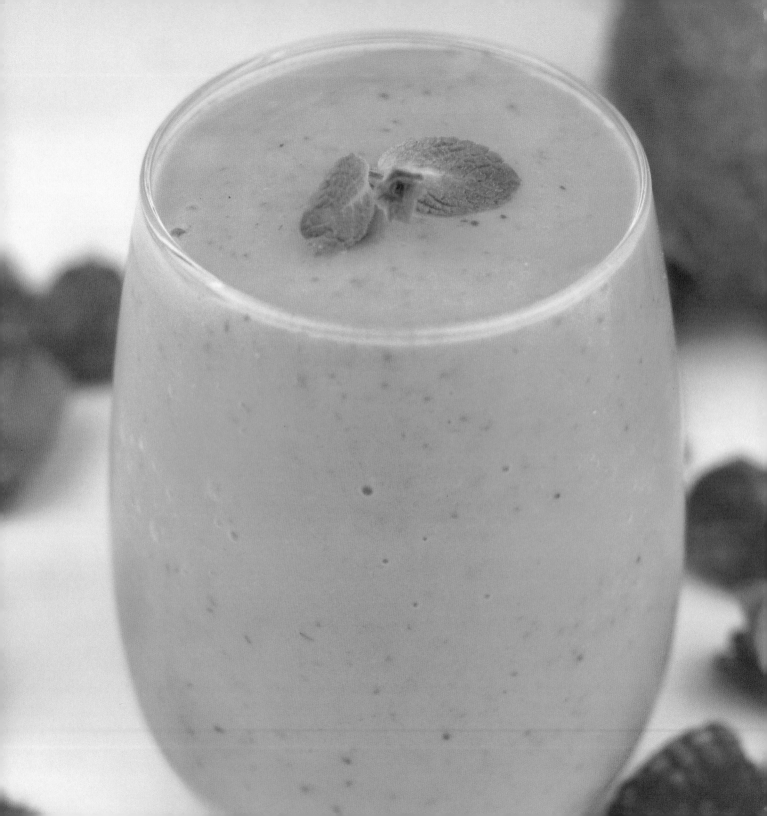

Mango Berries

This refreshing smoothie is loaded with antioxidants, nutrients, and vitamin C to help boost collagen production and keep skin glowing.

Instructions:

1. Place ingredients in a blender and purée until smooth.

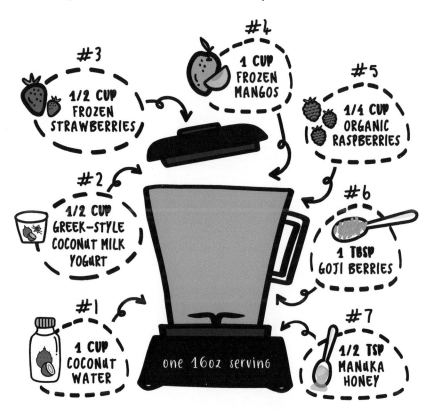

#3 1/2 CUP FROZEN STRAWBERRIES

#4 1 CUP FROZEN MANGOS

#5 1/4 CUP ORGANIC RASPBERRIES

#2 1/2 CUP GREEK-STYLE COCONUT MILK YOGURT

#6 1 TBSP GOJI BERRIES

#1 1 CUP COCONUT WATER

one 16oz serving

#7 1/2 TSP MANUKA HONEY

2. Pour into glass and serve immediately.

Ingredients:

1 Cup **Coconut Water**

1/2 Cup **Greek-Style Coconut Milk Yogurt (Plain or Vanilla Flavor)**

1/2 Cup **Frozen Strawberries**

1 Cup **Frozen Mangos**

1/4 Cup **Fresh Raspberries**

1 Tbsp **Goji Berries**

1/2 tsp **Manuka Honey**

HIGH ANTIOXIDANTS

Strawberries & Peaches

Ingredients:

1 1/2 Cups **Coconut Water**

1/2 Cup **Greek-Style Coconut Milk Yogurt (Plain or Vanilla Flavor)**

1 Cup **Frozen Strawberries**

3/4 Cup **Sliced Peaches**

1 Tbsp **Ground Flaxseed**

1/2 tsp **Manuka Honey**

Loaded with fiber and antioxidants, this refreshing smoothie is great for any party or just a self indulgence treat.

Instructions:

1. Place ingredients in a blender and purée until smooth.

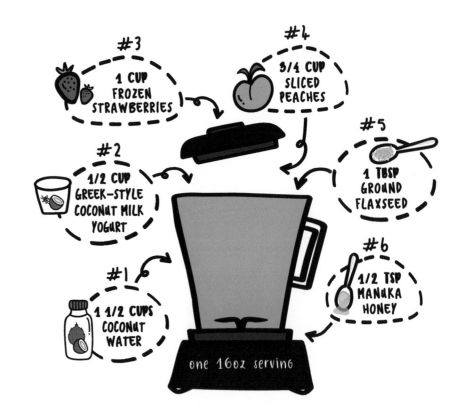

#3 1 CUP FROZEN STRAWBERRIES

#4 3/4 CUP SLICED PEACHES

#5 1 TBSP GROUND FLAXSEED

#2 1/2 CUP GREEK-STYLE COCONUT MILK YOGURT

#6 1/2 TSP MANUKA HONEY

#1 1 1/2 CUPS COCONUT WATER

one 16oz serving

2. Pour into glass and serve immediately.

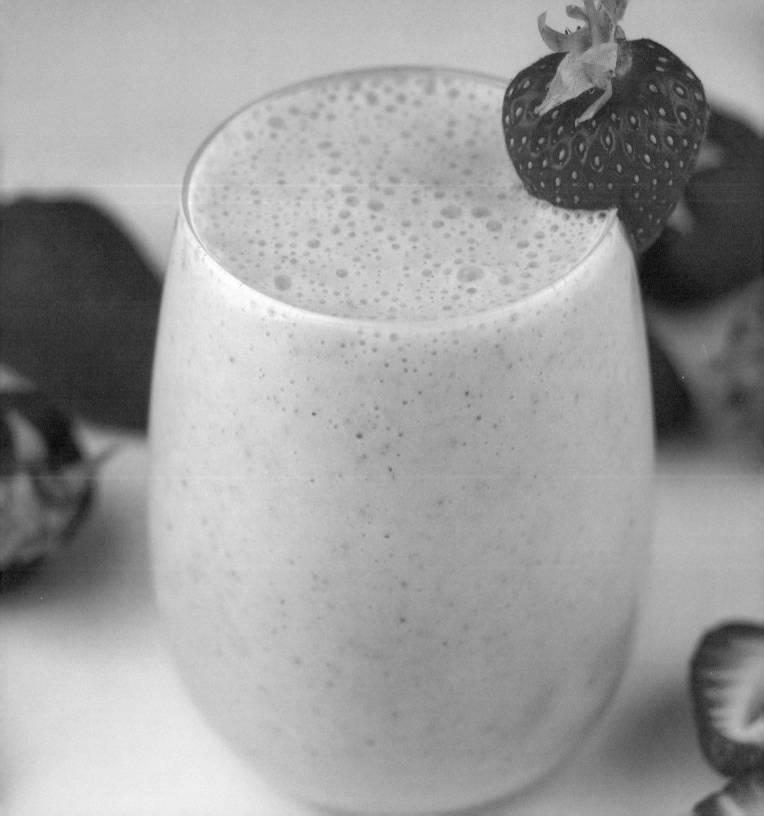

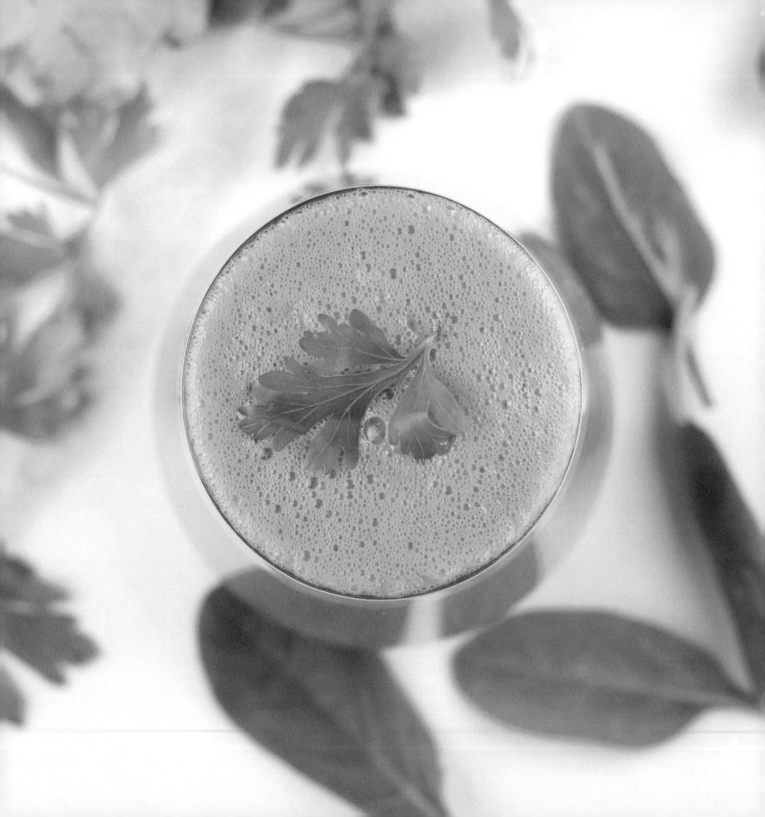

To all our readers, may these tips and recipes inspire you to blend your way to perfectly delicious smoothies and optimum health.

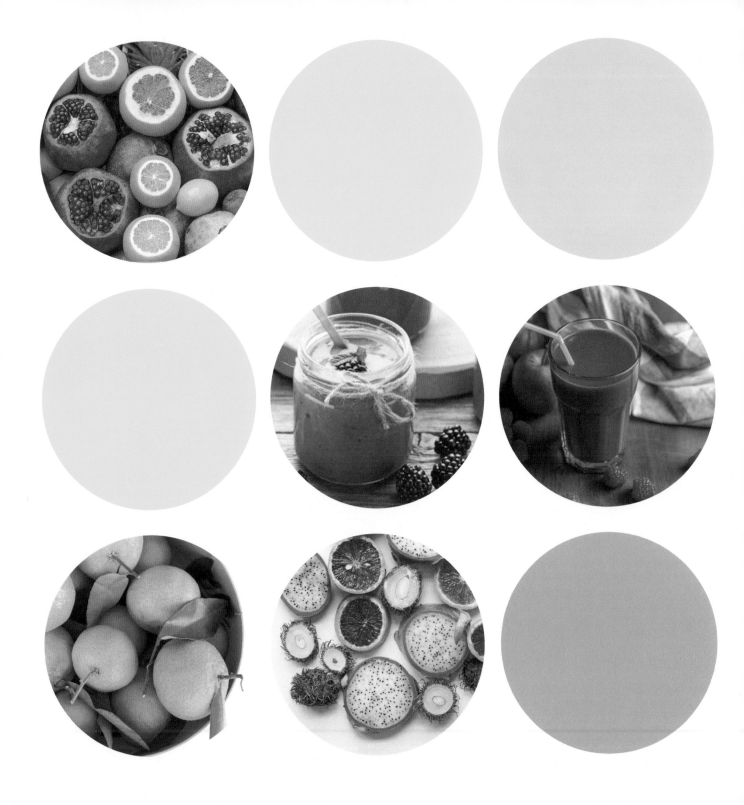

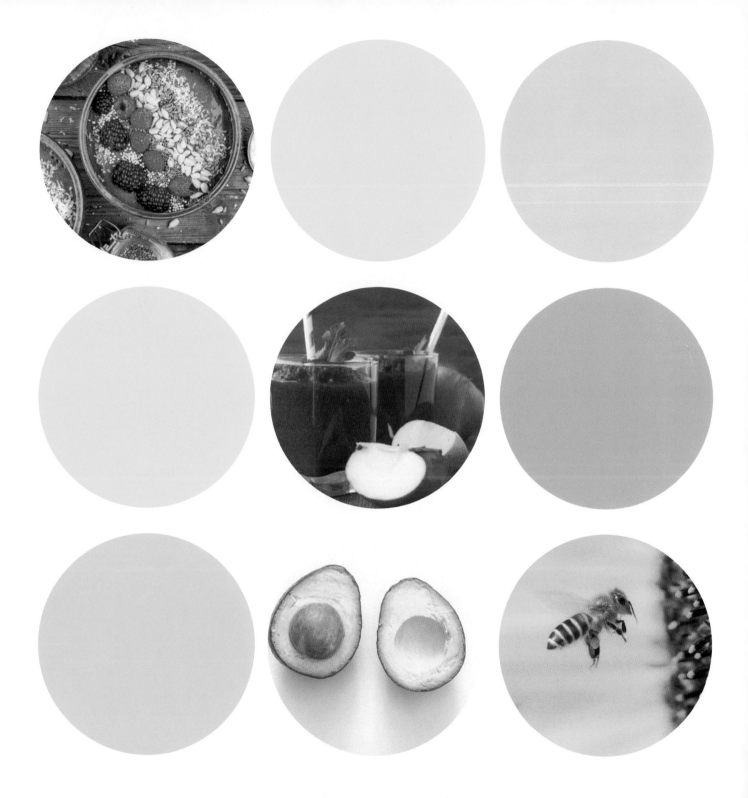

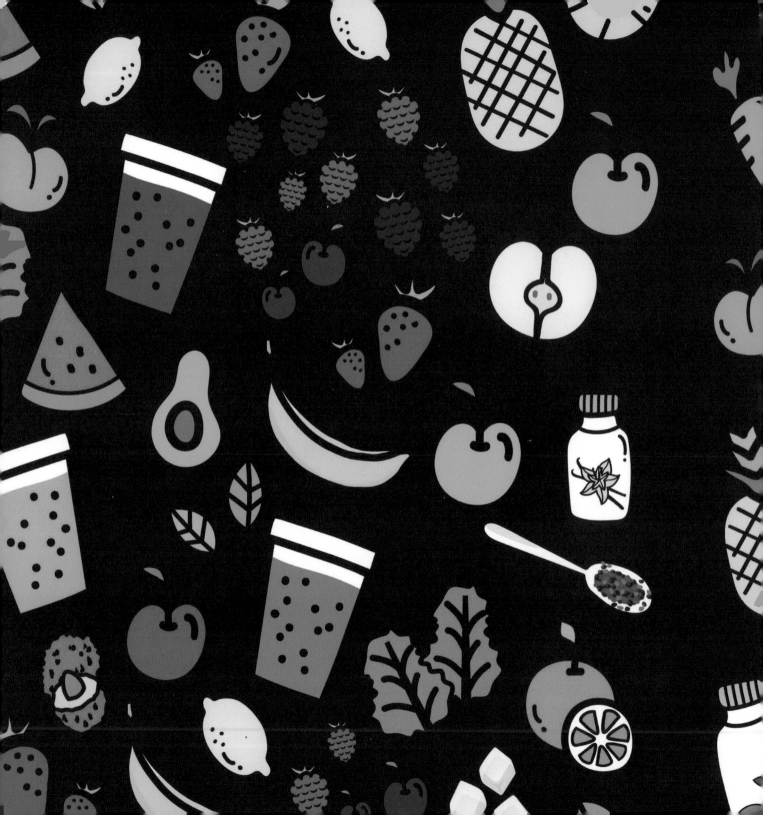

Printed in Great Britain
by Amazon

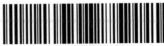